Aurum Manus®

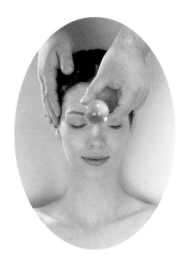

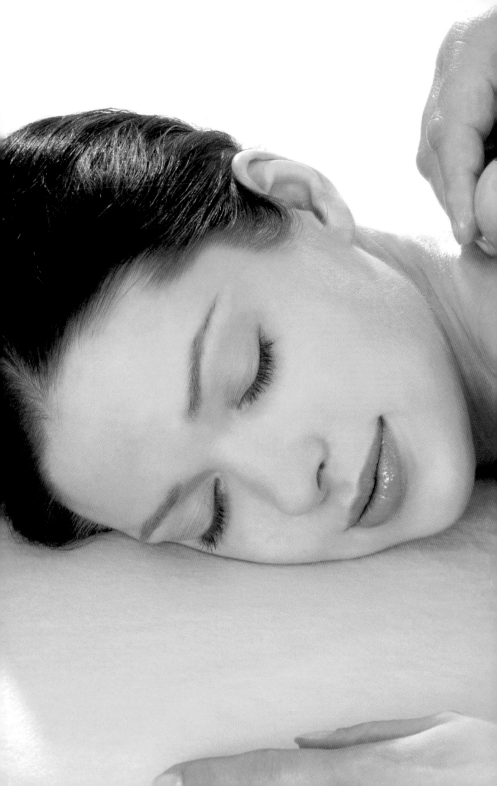

Ricky Welch

Aurum Manus®

The "Golden Hands" Method of
Crystal-based Holistic Massage

Contributions by
Iris Berg and
Michael Gienger

Photography by
Ines Blersch

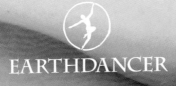

EARTHDANCER

A FINDHORN PRESS IMPRINT

Publisher's Note

The statements in this volume have been compiled according to the author's best knowledge and belief, and the healing effects of the crystals and massages described here have been tested many times over. As people can react in many different ways to treatment, the publisher and the author cannot provide any guarantee of the effectiveness or safety of the measures described herein. As in all cases of serious health problems and complaints, always please consult your physician or alternative therapist.

1 2 3 4 5 6 7 8 9 10 11 12 13 14 15 12 11 10 09 08 07 06

Aurum Manus®
Ricky Welch

Original German text © Ricky Welch
This English edition © 2006 Earthdancer GmbH
English translation © 2006 Astrid Mick

Title page photo: Ines Blersch
Design: Dragon Design, UK

Photographs: Ines Blersch, Stuttgart
Assistant: Jens Volle
Model: Stephanie and Peter
Hair / Makeup: Petra Ucakar, Stuttgart
Casting: fischercasting.de, Stuttgart

Edited by Stuart Booth

Typesetting and graphics: Dragon Design, UK
Typeset in ITC Garamond Condensed

Printed in China

ISBN-10: 1-84409-086-8
ISBN-13: 978-1-84409-086-0

Published by Earthdancer Books, an Imprint of:
Findhorn Press, 305a The Park, Findhorn, Forres IV36 3TE, Great Britain

Contents

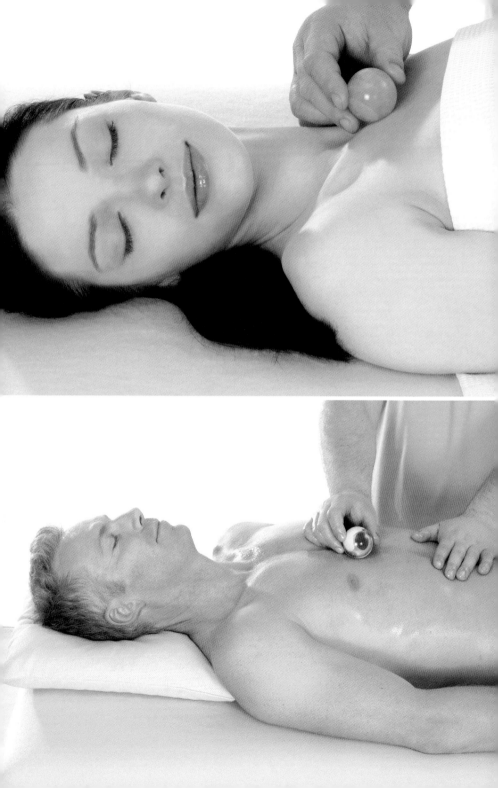

Golden Hands

A therapy that is able to treat tinnitus and migraines is, in itself, worth its weight in gold. If, at the same time, it is also a fantastically pleasurable experience, such as a massage by Ricky Welch, it becomes a veritable blessing for the body, soul and spirit.

In the spring of 2005, I experienced, for the first time, the great pleasure of an Aurum Manus® massage. Although I had been carrying out massage personally for 21 years, and had also had many massages, this treatment was something very special. An extremely pleasant combination of warmth, oil, flowing movements and gliding crystal spheres blew away all the stress from my bones and enveloped me as if in a cosy cocoon lasting for days afterwards. This was precisely the aspect of it all that surprised me most. I was frantically busy with a heavy workload during this period, rushing from one appointment to another. Yet, after the massage, I remained amazingly relaxed and unconcerned throughout and work seemed so much easier to perform. All too often we forget that expending all of one's energy can so often result in being neither effective nor having the hoped-for staying power, stamina, endurance, perseverance or persistence. Instead, it can so easily lead to an excess of pointless effort and use of our natural energies.

However, staying relaxed and worry-free during a period of great effort and stress does not just succeed any old how. Furthermore, even if we have actually recognised this fact, we first have to learn and then work on maintaining such an attitude. This is where the Aurum Manus® therapy is an enormous help. The massage techniques have been formulated in such a way that tension is rapidly reduced and the body remains unstressed.

Of course, holistically speaking, the body, the soul and the spirit are intimately connected. This is taken into account with the Aurum Manus® method, so that physical relaxation is extended quite naturally into a feeling of peace and spiritual calm. In fact, the Aurum Manus® concept goes even further in order that the resulting calm and tranquillity can be maintained via its sound nutritional advice, yoga and meditation exercises. These all help counteract the ever-present stress of modern life and help the recipient to create their own new life concept. In this way, along with due care and attention and a bit of time

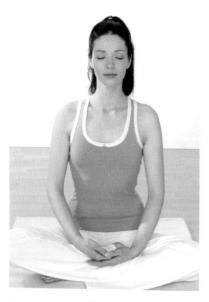

wonderful massage make such a beneficial "life change" far easier to achieve. Ricky's techniques and methods bestow an inner calm and give free range to our energies, both of which we need to master our lives.

The massage can make tinnitus, migraines, tension, back pain, joint problems and many other ailments and complaints seem to disappear, almost as a "side effect" of the treatment. Whether the complaints will disappear for good, however, depends very much upon the individual lifestyle, of course, and Aurum

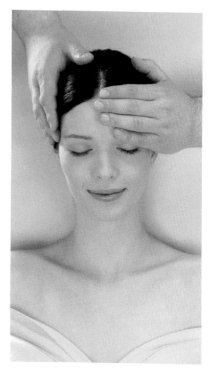

devoted to oneself, it is perfectly possible to become noticeably healthier, more stable and better balanced both psychologically and spiritually.

From my own experience, I can tell you it really is worth it! For forty years of my life, I worked flat out. Up until the point where I met Ricky Welch and the Aurum Manus® method and philosophy, I was a fully developed workaholic. I had realised this long before, but the concept of Aurum Manus® and its massage techniques were a great help in finally putting my "course correction" into practice. The very fact that Aurum Manus® is a way of keeping yourself healthy and balanced makes it particularly valuable.

Of course, Aurum Manus® is not the only therapy of its type. Nevertheless, the

Manus® makes no secret of this. But it does provide a vast amount of what is needed for a lasting life change. Even if its concepts are not entirely new or unknown to us, let's be completely honest: do we ever really put them into practice? For this reason alone, then, it is both useful and necessary to be reminded of the principles.

"*Aurum manus* - Golden hands!" was the spontaneous exclamation of a Latin teacher after a massage by Ricky Welch. Since then, many people have experienced and benefited from these golden hands, as Ricky has been treating and massaging tirelessly now for some 18 years. However, this book is meant to take this concept of "gold from the hands" even further, so that many other hands can, in future, touch and help in this same way and so the Aurum Manus® massage is the central theme of this book. Before that, though, Ricky tells us the remarkable story of his creation of the therapy. After a detailed outline of the techniques, the book concludes with further notes and advice on Aurum Manus® therapy.

I wish all its readers much pleasure, as well as an enhanced enjoyment of life. May you, too, take the gold contained herein into your hands!

Michael Gienger
Tübingen, autumn 2005

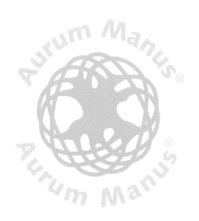

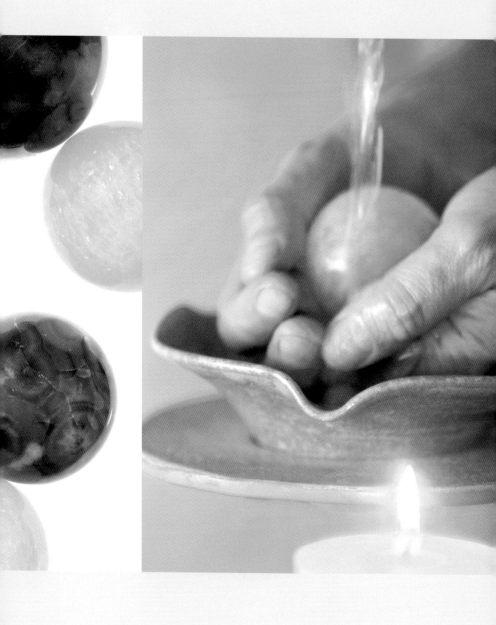

The Aurum Manus® Story

God sleeps in a stone,
Dreams in a plant,
Awakens in an animal
And acts in a human.
Hindu saying

The Initial Spark

It was during a work experience training session for swimming-pool lifeguards, at the tender age of thirteen, that I made a momentous decision. I was an enthusiastic swimmer at the time and a member of the DLRG (German Life-Savers Association) and was just taking my life-saving certificate. This included my needing to pass a practical unit by virtue of working as a lifeguard at the swimming pool during my summer holidays. It was during this period that I first experienced the techniques of massage – and I was deeply impressed! In fact, it was as if I had suddenly been transported to the "Arabian Nights": candles had been lit, there was the previously unexperienced but wonderful smell of aromatic oils, and the

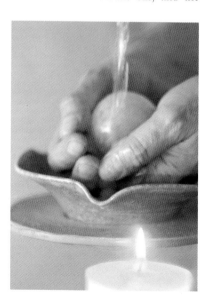

peace and quiet of the place was imbued with a magical atmosphere. Just like the young prince who is suddenly transported to fairyland, I stood there, gazing in astonishment. The beauty of this atmosphere took hold of me and touched me deeply. It was the moment I made my decision: I would become a masseur!

Having always been what I'd like to think of as "a man of action", I made my way to the School of Massage in Heidelberg as quickly as I could, in order to apply for a place on a course there. By chance, I arrived in the middle of the midday break. However, the head of the school, quite spontaneously, took twenty minutes to deal with me and my request. After all, it was hardly an everyday occurrence for a thirteen-year-old to march into the School of Massage, announcing: "I want to be a masseur!"

In fact, I was sent away with a friendly, but firm instruction: "Come back again in five years time!" – and so I found myself back out in the street and feeling rather disappointed. However, this in no way detracted from my decision and ambition in any way!

Therefore, first of all I finished school, for what was I to do? After that, I began an apprenticeship as a baker. This came to a premature end because I developed an allergy to the flour. Clearly, in just about every way, it was obviously not the right path for me.

When I was finally eighteen years old, I set out once more for the School of Massage. "Good morning, Mr. Welch!" the head greeted me as soon as I stepped into the room. I was amazed! Evidently, he had remembered the face and name of that thirteen-year-old over the years. Nevertheless, there was yet another disappointment in store for me: the training course, consisting of a maximum of 40 participants, was already fully subscribed!

Once again, I stood out in the street full of disappointment – but my decision still remained: I want to be a masseur! Then came what I still think of as a miracle. One week into the new training cycle, my telephone rang. It was the School of Massage: one student had unexpectedly dropped out and, if I could be available immediately, I could have his place. Of course, I could be there at once! If needs be, I would have left the telephone receiver hanging there in mid-air and dashed off to the School of Massage on the spot! Hallelujah!

Thus began my training as a masseur on 8 October 1988, a date that remains forever important to me.

The School of Massage was like paradise to me! Well, maybe not necessarily all the theoretical stuff, I have to admit, but the practical side of it was all the more exciting. I had a good, willing partner in Ingo Kieser, who shared my pas-

sion and was a heavenly masseur. What was tedious practice to others was bliss to us. It was true fulfilment – just trying out this or that movement... or would it not be better if one approached it like this... and so on.

From the very first day, we were unstoppable in our enthusiasm for experimentation, so that the days soon began and ended with the same old comments by my teacher, "Ah Welch, the first one again?" and "Right, Welch, time to go home!" But the end of the day was too soon for us, so we took our massage kits to the athletics and sports clubs and offered them our services. After all, what sporting type is likely to turn down the offer of a good massage? In this way, even during the first few weeks of our training, we managed to work on a number of footballers, wrestlers and weightlifters in order to try out our skills.

Our additional activities did not go unnoticed at the School of Massage, as I could not stop myself from sneaking in one or two of the hand movements that I had worked out myself. It seemed a sensible and natural thing to do, in fact. However, Mr Welzig, our teacher – and who always greeted everyone, somewhat ironically, with "Good day, professor" – seemed possessed of X-ray vision. He was able to spot, even across 20 massage tables, if a massage technique being applied was diverging from the authorised style or plan. Many were the times I would find him suddenly standing, saying: "Welch, what are you doing? We practise the Heidelberg massage here, not Shiatsu! I appreciate your thirst for knowledge knows no bounds, but stick to this: one step after the other!"

Of course he was right! Mr Welzig was, and always remains, one of my idols. He was always calm and collected, a first-rate teacher, whom one could emulate and, as a masseur, he had what I can only describe as "golden hands". For me, he is the very "Father of Massage". Through him, I realised that it was only sensible to learn *every* type of massage, very thoroughly in its own right, and to improve my technique continuously. Nevertheless, he had dropped in an interesting key word – "Shiatsu". What was it and where did it come from, I wondered? Had I involuntarily discovered something that already existed elsewhere? As a typical eighteen-year-old, I wanted to know straightaway and not at some time in the future. In fact, my answer was to come soon, but in a most unexpected way...

A Triumph of Impudence

On the 8 December 1988, just two months after my training as a masseur had begun, the famous Scorpions rock band came to give a concert in Eppelheim. Of course, I did not want to miss this and made my way to the evening ticket office.

Imagine my disappointment to find out that the concert was sold out. I was dismayed. There I stood, in the rain, but not in the least bit inclined to give up yet. Somehow or other I was going to get into the gig. There is some Irish blood in my veins which gives me a certain stubbornness and persistence, and so I simply had to find a way to get in.

Suddenly, I had an idea! I ran back to my car, threw on my white coat and grabbed my portable massage table and my ever-ready case of massage equipment. Armed with all this, I made a beeline for the backstage entrance, in front of which, naturally, stood the usual human security barrier.

"Hello, I'm the masseur!" I said in as relaxed a tone as I could muster – and in spite of sweating palms, I tried to remain cool.

"Whose masseur?" was the less than encouraging answer of the six-foot-tall bodyguard. "Well, I don't know – somebody here ordered a masseur," I said.

Suspicious eyes gave me the once over.

"Well, I suppose you'd better come with me, then."

Thus, promisingly, the door opened and I went in. The object of my desire seemed to be in sight. However, my path was to prove more like one through Hell and I was about to pay for my con trick pretty quickly.

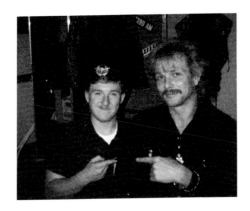

I had imagined it all rather differently: I was going to overcome the entry problem with the "massage trick", and then they would find out that nobody had booked a masseur. Then I would say that, since I was now in and had come over specially, if I could just stay for the concert. Then, of course, they were bound to give me a seat. An ingenious idea, wasn't it? That's what I thought, but it all turned out very differently!

The fact that things were not running to plan became apparent the moment the bodyguard took me to the Scorpions manager. He caught sight of me and flipped.

"What's this? What does he want?"

I shrank down to a few inches (with my hat!) and could not speak one word, so the security guy answered for me.

"He says we ordered a masseur."

"Ordered a masseur? Who ordered a masseur? Nobody here ordered a mas-

seur!" came the thunderous retort.

Ouch! This was not looking good. Better to beat a hasty retreat.

"Well then, please excuse me," I said in a small voice. "I'd better go then."

Let me get out of here as fast as possible, I thought.

Then the trap snapped shut!

"You're not going anywhere," the manager thundered on, "before I've found out what's going on here!"

Now I was really scared! "Jesus," I thought, "this is sure to be the end of my short career as a masseur. If this gets out, I'll be chucked out of the school, nobody else will take me on, and I will never be a masseur. Then I suppose I'll have to knead dough again and cough over the flour dust, or... or?"

I felt sick and dizzy. Pictures popped into my head of me being arrested, standing in front of the head of the School, being expelled, etc., scenes of my future failed life. A life wasted forever. I broke out in a sweat. All I wanted was to get away from there.

However, maybe it is the cases that God punishes small sins on the spot. The investigations went on.

"Who ordered a masseur here?" the manager roared at everybody in general.

Everyone shook their heads and there were puzzled expressions all round. Things were getting serious. I felt like a rabbit in a trap. Then, suddenly and unexpectedly, help arrived. A friendly woman called Tootsie appeared, calmed the manager - who had gradually turned from an avenging angel into a raging fury - and promised to sort out the matter. Maybe one of the musicians had ordered a masseur?

They hadn't, but Rudolph Schenker, one of the Scorpions' guitarists, was delighted when he heard that a masseur was present.

"Fantastic!" he said, "I've had this backache ever since I jumped down from a speaker just now. Bring the man to me!"

Suddenly, nobody was asking where the heck I had come from anymore, and soon there I was unfolding my massage table. But it was not over yet.

Hardly had I started the massage when I realised why he had backache. When he had jumped down from the loudspeaker, two of his vertebrae had slipped. But pushing back vertebrae was strictly forbidden to massage students. What should I do? The noose was closing tightly on me again. Should I push the vertebrae back in place? What if something went wrong? Once again, images of my departure from the School of Massage reeled before my inner eye. But there was no turning back! After all, here in my hands was a person suffering pain, who shortly had to perform an exhausting two-hour concert. So, I pushed aside my fears and worries and gave the massage my very best shot! Lo and behold, the backache had disappeared after the massage. Schenker was overwhelmed.

"That was the best massage I have ever had!" he told me.

At last my adrenalin levels could gradually subside and my seat in the concert was a certainty. I was even beginning to relax sufficiently in order to enjoy it somewhat. However, when the show was finally over, I packed up my gear as quickly as I could and fled during all the fuss backstage.

Wow, what a story! I was so relieved to have escaped again, but naturally also rather proud of my adventure. This was why I could not stop myself from telling it all to my friends and some fellow students at the School next day. I was really made up and felt good.

It didn't last for long, though. That very same day, I was told, "Ricky, they're looking for you!"

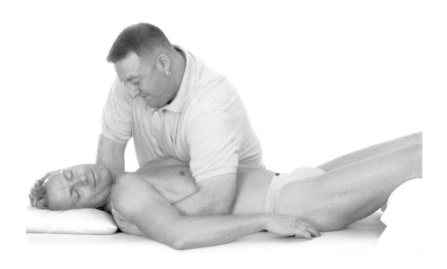

The local radio station was saying that the Scorpions were looking for the masseur from the evening before. I began to panic. Was it all going to come out after all? What did they want me for? If only I had kept my mouth shut, I could have stayed "under cover". This was why everybody now knew about the episode. Consequently, I thought it would be better if I went and owned up before somebody blew the whistle and they came to me. So, for the third time, with knees knocking, I went out from the School of Massage and along to the hotel where the Scorpions were staying.

There I was greeted in a much friendlier manner than I had been the night before.

"Why did you just disappear?" the manager asked me. "We owe you money for your treatment."

What! Why? What for? I was speechless. They were not going to sue me, after all! It was all about my fee! At this point, my guilty conscience would not let me rest, and I decided to make a full and frank confession!

Naturally, this ensured a great deal of merriment among the band and the management. However, the upshot was that I got my first professional engagement, right there and then. After just two months at the School of Massage, I was the Scorpions' official masseur!

For the next eight years, I accompanied the band on its tours. It was an appointment that turned out to be probably the most important one of my life. At least, Aurum Manus®, in its present form, would never have existed otherwise.

Many Paths, Many Teachers

I travelled all over the world with the Scorpions. Of course, in the beginning, it was rather difficult to fit it all in with my training at the School of Massage. I definitely had to, and wanted to, finish the course. But, whenever possible, I joined the band on tour in order to ply my trade as their masseur. The dark rings under my eyes became a little more prominent during that time, and the theoretical part of my course also suffered somewhat. Nevertheless, my great interest lay in practising the art of massage and, in truth, nothing better could have happened than the job with the Scorpions.

Thanks to the many tours all over the world, I was able to meet a number of massage teachers in a variety of cultures and traditions. No matter in what country we happened to be, I would always use the opportunity to undertake extra training in the local massage schools. In my free time, I would hunt out massage centres and schools and ask if I might watch the masseurs at work there. The information that I was the Scorpions' official masseur usually opened all doors to me pretty rapidly.

"Come on in" is what I was usually told and soon we would be immersed in an exchange on massages, techniques, hand positions, effects and so on. I was even able to benefit by simply watching, so I could "feel" and experience just how effective a particular massage technique could be as soon as I saw it. In this way I learned Shiatsu, Thai massage, oriental massage, Lomi Lomi Nui, Turkish Hamam massage, Ayurvedic massage and a number of other things from the masters of the art in their own cultural context. I was so happy, and things could not have been better! In this way, gradually, I was able to build up my own, wide-ranging massage repertoire.

Contacts with other rock bands were also forged as my reputation gradually began to spread. I undertook massage sessions on band members of U2, AC/DC, Roxette and Gianna Nannini among others – using ever more feeble excuses to creep away from the School of Massage to attend the concerts. Although my teachers turned a blind eye (or two) because of my proven practical skills, the theoretical side of my training began to sink to a level of what was barely tolerable. As a result, I was forced to curb my extra-curricular activities somewhat until I had finally finished my studies. After that, nothing could hold me back and massage became my whole life.

Doing It My Way

After eight years "on tour", I had also become tired of all the travelling and so left the Scorpions in order to open up my own massage practice. The break was not an easy one for me, though, and I still

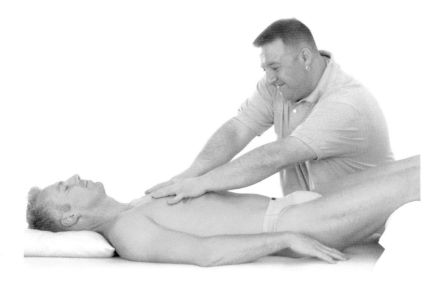

maintain friendly relations with the band members.

However, it was high time for me to go my own way. I was beginning to feel that I wanted to create a unified system of massage derived from the many elements I had learned about during those eight years. Of course, I also wanted to find out what could be achieved with such a form of massage and the permanence and stability of my own practice was the only real way of making this happen.

I continued to refine the sequence of the techniques that I employed in massage sessions, developing my own hand movements and abandoning some of the concepts I had learned at the School of Massage. I had also discovered pretty quickly that people immersed in modern Westernised culture have what I can only describe as too much energy in their

heads. Because of this, it is unsuitable and inappropriate to massage the front of the body from the feet up to the head – as I had learned at the School, but also in some of the Eastern massage techniques – as the energy build-up in the head simply increases that way.

With this in mind, I tried out working in the opposite direction, and massaged the front of the body from the head down to the feet. The results were self-evident and many clients thanked me for the "best massage they had ever had". In addition, it was also clear that the effects of the massage lasted far longer.

A further important aspect of my developing technique was recognising the basic principle of always "maintaining the flow" while massaging. The concept, which came from the East, that a constant stream of energy flows through the body made me realise that any interruption of the massage could also result in an interruption in this flow of energy. Stopping for a moment to replenish the massage oil, changing sides or moving to another area of the body are all interruptions that probably detract from the required state of relaxation. Thus I began to work "in a single flow", one hand always remaining on the client's body, and with changeovers conducted in a fluid manner. Essentially, this involves first one hand making contact with a different area of the body before the second leaves the previous one. In this way, the massage of one side of the body remains one of a single, flowing contact. The proof of the technique's soundness was that my clients simply could not get enough of it – and this confirmed that I was on the right track.

Warm massage oil – copious quantities of which are used, for example, in Ayurvedic massage from India – became a further important component of my sessions. Using the right kind of oil, massage treatments can be better targeted. This is why I employ only high-grade, organic oils during massage. Combined with the correct movements and holds on the body, warm oil also makes it possible to obtain a truly deep state of relaxation. Indeed, it takes over a greater part of the actual work involved.

The next step for me was the discovery of using crystals in massage. These days, I cannot even imagine working without them, but they came into play almost by accident. This is what happened.

I used to employ wooden massage tools, as they are used as part of Eastern massage techniques, in order to stimulate certain pressure points or to move along the meridians (the energy channels) of the body. The problem with these wooden rods is that over time they become brittle through use and may even splinter. Naturally, this is extremely unpleasant for the client if one is working with a certain amount of pressure along a meridian when the wood splinters. One day I was about to carry out a massage in which I normally used these small rods but, after checking them, I realised they were definitely no longer suitable for the job. I rushed off to the Chinese retailer from whom I had always obtained them in the past. I just managed to get there before closing time. Alas, they were all sold out. A new delivery was due some time, but I needed the rods at once as the session was booked that same day, and I could not go back without the implements. However, my resourceful Chinese retailer had a suggestion – and handed me a few small pieces of jade. "These stones will help for the time being!" he said. Puzzled, and a trifle sceptical, I went on my way. Use crystals for a massage? Well, better than nothing, I supposed...

The pieces of jade were *considerably* better than nothing! Even during the first massage using them, I realised that something rather special was going on. Even the difficult, tense areas of the client's body seemed to relax a little faster than when working with the wooden rods. Or was this impression just an illusion, I wondered to myself? In order to be sure, I used the crystals on several different clients and there was definitely a positive response.

I pondered further upon this. Maybe, after all, it was no accident that jade was considered to be a sacred crystal in China - the land of acupuncture and acupressure. At any rate, the little wooden rods were forgotten for the time being, and I dedicated myself to investigating the jade crystals.

However, for the clients, the crystals I used for massage proved to feel unpleasantly cold in their normal state - so I simply placed them in the pre-warmed massage oil to warm them up before use. Doing this, I found that not only did they then feel much better on the skin but they also provided an extra means of retaining warmth and intrinsic energy, before I gradually re-released them. Indeed, my clients soon made it clear that they greatly preferred these warmed crystals.

Therefore, over time, this was how my massage methods evolved - using warm

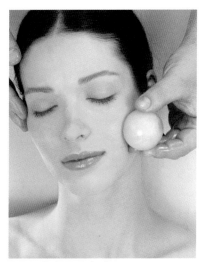

Jade crystal sphere massage

oil and warmed crystals, together with my own technique of a flowing sequence of hand movements. It was my personal creation, and "Ricky's Massage" quickly gained a highly favourable reputation.

Tinnitus and Migraine

Nevertheless, in those early days, I still had no idea what was yet to come! The decisive turning point, which was to lead to Aurum Manus®, did not occur until 1999.

At the time, I was the head of the Binshof Thermal Spa in Speyer. There too, I had established a flourishing massage business, using my special techniques, and was busily occupied with it. During that period, I was visited by a friend who suffered from truly bad migraines. The attacks would recur again and again after only short intervals of relief and each attack, literally, laid him low. Naturally, he had seen a doctor regularly and had gone from one clinic to another, as well as having tried various therapies. But it had been all to no avail. It really pained me, both personally and professionally, to watch helplessly, yet I had no idea what to do about his migraines. I thought long and often about how I might help my friend. Then, one day, a complete stranger gave me the following advice: "You should pray!"

Now, while I would not consider myself a bad person, I was certainly not one of the most religiously pious ones either! Praying was not exactly "my thing". Still, one day, while driving and wondering yet again about my friend's hopeless situation, I suddenly found myself exclaiming: "You up there, if you really exist, then help my friend!"

Of course, like many people, I had some kind of basic idea in my head that if God really existed, why could he not simply make things happen "as if by magic". However, the reality is apparently rather different, as we too have a part to play and must contribute to the realising of our wishes. I had no inkling of this at the time, and certainly not in this particular context. Indeed, it would never have occurred to me that I might actually become precisely the person who would be able to help my friend.

However, shortly after this "prayer", if that is what it was, I had the same dream twice in succession. In my dream, I saw myself treating certain parts of a face with the same hand movements each time. In particular, the point between the eyebrows appeared to play a special role in this treatment.

Initially, I took little or no notice of this dream. However, when it occurred for the *third* time, I began to take it more seriously. Then my training in Asian medical techniques began to bear fruit. When I repeated the hand movements from the dream on the same points, but in a waking state, I suddenly understood that I was dealing with meridians - the very same acupuncture points of traditional Chinese medicine and the so-called "third eye", another important energy centre recognised in the same medical tradition. The same location is also called the "brow chakra" in Ayurvedic medicine (*chakra* is originally from Sanskrit, meaning "wheel". Among other meanings, too, it also refers to our own revolving energy centres. The question was clear to me: could this dream be an answer to the question I had been turning over for so long?

So we tried it out. I massaged my friend with this "dream-created" technique - and it actually worked! Not only did the migraine attacks decrease in intensity, the intervals between such attacks became longer and longer. Furthermore, my friend's problem with tinnitus disappeared too.

This feedback surprised me personally, as I was unaware that he had also been suffering from these persistent and annoying rushing noises in the ear. During our friendship of many years, he had only ever spoken about his migraines and never mentioned the tinnitus. The fact that the migraines had actually improved made me so very happy that, initially, I paid no attention to the healing of the tinnitus problem. So, naturally, I adopted this newly "discovered" massage technique and used it in my programme, calling it a "regeneration massage" - especially where severe tension and exhaustion coincided, and it turned out to be a real blessing for my clients.

I did not return to the subject of tinnitus until much later. One day, a well-known German female singer came to me for a massage at the Binshof Spa.

The "dreamed" energy points

Basically, and not to denigrate her in any way, she was what is often dubbed a "power rock chick". However, she had decided to take a lengthy "artistic break" at the time.

Then, during the massage sessions, I discovered that the reason for her break was a severe bout of tinnitus, which had been tormenting her for about four years. Maybe too much amplified, on-stage volume, who can tell? However, the keyword "tinnitus" reminded me of my "dream-created" treatment once again. So I incorporated it into the session with her.

After the massage, she seemed somewhat distracted in her conversation. She moved her head back and forth, as if she were looking for something. Yes, lo and behold, the tinnitus had disappeared! And while it did return, this sudden interruption, after four years of constant 'noise', made her feel very hopeful. We arranged further appointments and, after the eighth massage session, the tinnitus was finally gone for good!

Well, the word got around. Within a short time, more and more people suffering from tinnitus turned up at my practice and made appointments. In many cases, though not in all, I confess, the massage really did result in improvements.

Doctors who were treating these same people for the condition became curious about the unexpected results. It was in this way that my first real contacts with the medical profession were established.

In fact, by a wonderful coincidence, it just so happened that the South West German radio station SWR was conducting interviews at the hotel attached to the Binshof Spa, asking guests how they liked it there. I happened to be passing and was also asked.

"Oh, I really like it here, I work here!" was my answer, and soon I was chatting to the reporter. We talked about the massage facility at the spa, about my work and about much more. All of this resulted in the reporter actually having one of my massages as part of his story, while his colleagues recorded the conversation during my hands-on session.

Suddenly, and without prior discussion, he put the following question to me: "I understand you also treat tinnitus and migraines here? While this was not quite correct, expressed in such terms – as I am neither a doctor nor an alternative therapist, not actually treating illnesses but simply providing massages – it was nonetheless broadcast in that way. As a consequence, my appointments diary was completely overwhelmed. The Binshof Spa was swamped by clients wanting massages, many of who were hoping for relief from tinnitus and migraines. It was just too much! I was a mere masseur and did not want to play the part of a doctor. Consequently, I was on the brink of beating a hasty retreat from the sudden fame.

The Birth of Aurum Manus®

However, Fate, or whatever, had other plans for me. Through this radio broadcast and reports by patients, and especially those by a well-known German rock singer, the Tinnitus League (a self-help organisation for sufferers) had become aware of me. Was this possibly an effective tinnitus therapy? It had to be investigated!

This was how contact came about with Dr Lindenberger of the Schwetzingen Hospital near Heidelberg. He invited me for a chat and I drove there, without any references or presentation. Quite simply, I explained to him what had happened, and how I had, basically, stumbled into this whole field of therapy for tinnitus and migraines.

Luckily, Dr Lindenberger was truly interested! Together with Dr von Renmont – of the pressure chamber centre, where many patients with severe tinnitus problems are treated – a study was begun to investigate the effectiveness of my massage methods.

Over a period of some five years, from 1999 to 2004, the doctors in the group around Dr Lindenberger and Dr von Renmont sent a total of 133 tinnitus patients to me for treatment. All had been first examined by doctors and many of them had already undergone all the known traditional medical treatments. Such procedures ranged from infusions to treatment in a pressure chamber, all without notable success.

I was definitely not dealing with the "easy cases" only. Nevertheless, in more than half of the patients, a clear improvement was obvious. Furthermore, in many cases, there was actually a complete cessation of the noises in the patients' ears. For many of them, who were suffering constantly from what they called "internal noise", this was a sheer and unbelievable relief!

These positive results were confirmed by subsequent medical examinations and thereby ensured a validity and basic trust in my treatment that was destined to grow – and, unusually, but satisfyingly, it was from the recommendations of the traditional medical establishment itself.

At the same time, in dealing specifically with tinnitus and migraine patients, I was able to further refine and improve my treatment's techniques. Everything that I had learned up to that point now seemed to merge within me. Indeed, a new form of massage emerged that was a mix of my "dream-created" basic method and the subsequent wealth of practical experience. Even though my massage methods had long before become holistic in terms of an overall philosophy, something that was much more than the sum of the parts had been established. Any gaps that I had hitherto seemed to have, in spite of my vision and experience, had now been filled using my basic intuition.

I put this down almost entirely to the fact that, by this time, I had begun integrating the use of more and more crystals into my treatments. Oddly, at this point, I had actually not read any of the widespread literature that is available on healing crystals. However, the idea of not merely using jade, but integrating other crystals into my treatments, had occurred to me before.

It was very basic; I simply saw certain crystals and had the intrinsic feeling that I should try them out as part of my treatments. Therefore it was a real vindication

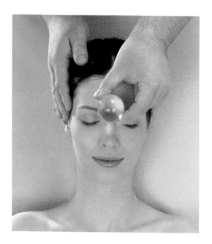

of such intuition when every attempt, involving new minerals, led to another small success!

Jade, rose quartz and citrine were the first ones that I tried, but were soon followed by rock crystal, mookaite, dumortierite and several others.

It also became clear to me that some crystals showed better results if in a cool state (i.e. at room temperature) rather than if they had been warmed first. Cool rock crystal placed around the eyes, for example, is simply heavenly in feel and effect!

Thus my range of massage methods grew and became a clearly identified and unique set of techniques. So it seemed to be the time to give the "child" a name.

A techno-medical term such as "massage for tinnitus and migraine according to Ricky Welch" was so clumsy as to be totally out of the question. Rather, I

wanted a name that would actually express the experience of the massage itself. Then I recalled quite suddenly a scene from at least a decade earlier. A Latin teacher had just got up from my massage table. Overcome by the feeling of relief the experience had given him, he exclaimed, "*Aurum manus*! – You have hands of gold!"

That was it: *Aurum manus*, "gold from the hands", just had to be the name of this new kind of massage. Both the experience and the effect of the massage were both encapsulated in the picture that this name conjured up. There was simply no better name. Thus the foundation stone was laid for the Aurum Manus® therapy, to which I now wish to introduce you in the pages of this book.

New Perspectives

The following few years were quite incredible. I could barely escape the turmoil and upheaval that threatened to overwhelm me completely on more than one occasion. Through a number of different television broadcasts, Aurum Manus® became known in about fifteen different countries. In Germany alone, three separate television reports were dedicated to accounts of this new therapy: on SAT 1 in 2001; in a programme called "Brisant" on MDR in 2002; and on SAT1 again in 2003. In the latter, Dr Lindenberger of Schwetzingen Hospital even

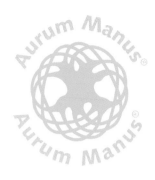

stated that the Aurum Manus® therapy was "of greater effectiveness than traditional medicine".

Ever since then, the cost of Aurum Manus® therapy has actually been reimbursed to clients by some medical insurance schemes, such has been its reputation, and depending on the individual cases and doctor's notes.

Nevertheless, this television programme led to me suffering a complete breakdown. The telephone rang constantly, and in one month alone I received 40,000 e-mail messages. I could no longer cope with it all. Something had to be done!

It became clear to me that I would first have to train other masseurs and therapists in order to meet the obvious demand for treatment. It pained me considerably not to be able to answer the many, many requests personally – but there it was.

Of course, as a masseur, I have only one pair of hands. How could I ever hope to help all these people? Well, clearly I could not. What was needed were more hands, more people who had the right

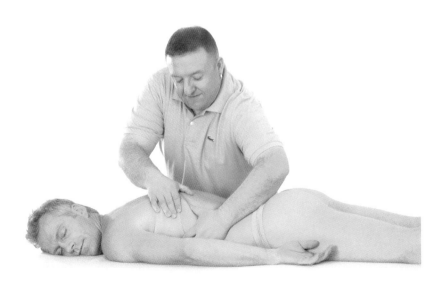

attitude, who would learn the Aurum Manus® therapy and then apply it.

I began to train my first students and supervisors and, during 2004, developed a close working relationship with the therapist Iris Berg from Karlsruhe-Durlach. Iris and I were a strong team right from the start, and Iris now heads the Aurum Manus® training courses in Germany. In the meantime, many more therapists – male and female – have completed their training, so that we now feel able to take the next step and introduce the Aurum Manus® therapy to an even wider public by means of this book.

However, this book also has another purpose. The Aurum Manus® massage, in spite of its great effectiveness, is actually quite simple and is based upon relaxation massage techniques that, once understood, can be carried out by just about anybody. This is real "hands on" proof of the old saying that states there is truth in simplicity.

In fact, I had toyed for some time with the idea of putting Aurum Manus® massage at the disposal of all in book form. My thinking was that if it were indeed true that, in Germany alone, millions of people suffer from tinnitus and migraines then this massage should be open to all who wished to take advantage of its curative results. Naturally, learning massage is best done on a practical basis, which is why we continue to offer courses and training programmes.

Nevertheless, anyone with the right degree of sympathy and a certain sensitivity, or who has already learned massage, should be able to take from this book the essence of all that they need to know about the method. The descriptions, based upon my many years experience are accompanied by Ines Blersch's beautiful photographs, which contribute a great deal towards making the massage principles and techniques that much clearer.

Just when I was "pregnant" with the idea for this book, I suddenly discovered – on 8 December 2004, in a Speyer bookshop – a recently published book entitled *Edelstein-Massagen* ("Massage with Crystals").

So it appeared that there really were already other masseurs using crystals in their work and there I had been working away at it myself for year! I purchased the book, rushed home and picked up the telephone.

The book was by Michael Gienger and I was lucky enough to be able to speak to him there and then. As I now know, I had caught him in the middle of a highly stressful stage of his life – which was why he explained to me, in a friendly, but very firm manner, that he had absolutely no time to talk at that moment. I was just about to say goodbye, but managed to include two or three muttered sentences about massaging with crystals, about tinnitus and migraines. The nature and atmosphere of the conversation changed instantly. In a trice, we both had our diaries to hand and made an appointment to meet up on the following Monday, 13 December 2004.

The moment we met we both felt that our encounter was really meant to be. Michael Gienger turned out to be an expert on minerals and crystal healing with 20 years' experience, as well as being an enthusiastic masseur who used Shiatsu and crystals. It was clear to me immediately that we would soon be pooling our experiences, as we both shared the desire to help people and to pass on this very important knowledge to others.

This is why I am extremely pleased that Michael is so closely involved in the publication of this book. Our acquaintance long ago turned into friendship, and massage using crystals is now taking us on old and new paths.

We invite you all to join us on this journey.

Ricky Welch
Altlussheim, summer 2005

Do not let someone you meet feel unhappy after their encounter with you.

Mother Teresa

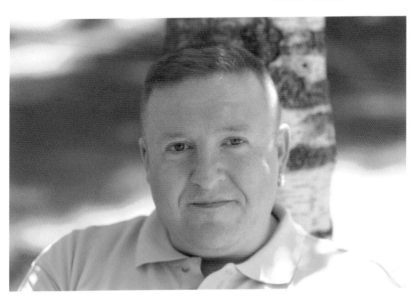

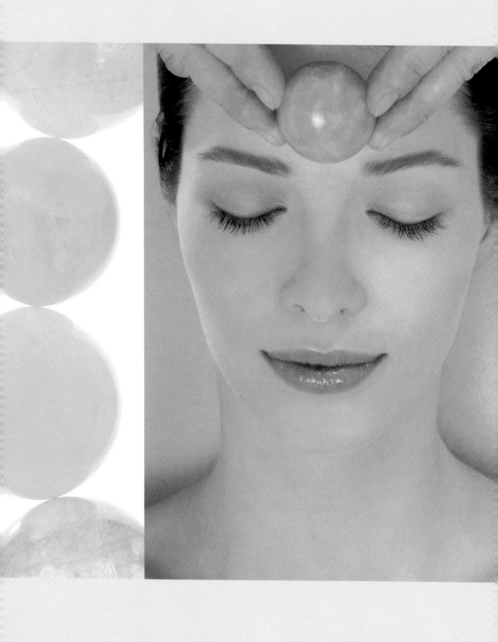

The Aurum Manus® Massage

My hand is God.
Endlessly blissful is my hand.
This hand safeguards all healing secrets,
Which make things whole, with its gentle touch.
                                        Rigveda

The word "massage" derives from the Arabic *massa,* "to touch". It is probably the oldest form of therapy in the world. The realisation that the correct type of touch can be healing is known in all cultures without exception. As a result, well-known forms and refined systems of massage have evolved in many traditions over thousands of years. Consider, for example, the Ayurveda, the ancient healing art of India or the acupuncture of China, a tradition that is at least four thousand years old. In Europe, and throughout the West too, there is the Graeco-Roman tradition of massage with a history going back several millennia. Therefore, in talking about massage, it is important to be aware of this historical context.

For thousands of years, various different massage techniques have survived – mainly thanks to being passed on orally from one generation to the next. Some survived in secret for centuries, being known only within individual families or secret lodges. In ancient Egypt, around 4000 BCE, for example, it was only certain

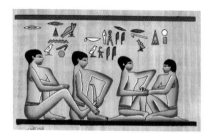

priests and priestesses who were initiated into the high art of massage.

In other places, insights into the healing effects of massage were gained in rather unusual ways. The Indian Marmar pressure points were actually developed around 6000 years ago on battlefields in order to inflict death – until it was discovered that there were certain points on the body which, if pressed gently and persistently, led to healing.

Around 2300 BCE, the Chinese perfected massage techniques involving acupressure. Together with the physical movement exercises of Tai Chi, careful nutrition and mental training (meditation), the Eastern concepts of holistic human health emerged very early on. In those days, one did not wait until an "unbalanced" condition had arisen. Instead, efforts to seek a preventative cure would have been made in order to "prevent" the lack of balance even developing. The word cure comes from the Latin *cura,* meaning "care", "looking after" and "welfare".

In European antiquity, too, we can already trace a refined curative system, which may well be said to have been ahead of our present knowledge in some respects. There are plenty of well-preserved Roman baths still in existence from which one can easily imagine how much spiritual and emotional pleasure was involved in overall ideas of human well-being. This was all part of what we now term a holistic approach in order to restore one's mind, body and spirit to a state of overall harmony. This concept of "natural medicine" then rapidly evolved during a period of about 1200 years, spreading throughout Europe with Graeco-Turkish massage and steam baths, reflexology, use of herbs and healing plants, Arabian alchemy and crystal healing. By the twelfth century, the saintly Hildegard von Bingen (1098–1179) had already developed holistic healing practices by combining many of these elements. It was an art in which, for example, crystal therapy had an important place.

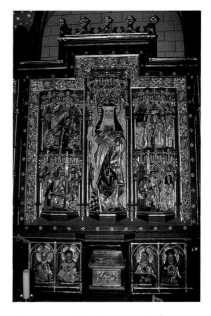

Thus the self-same application of crystals reintroduced via Aurum Manus® therapy can be traced back to European antiquity. Even the Greek and Roman lapidaries of Theophrastus and Pliny, for example, list the healing properties of certain crystals. Later, in the Middle Ages and in addition to Hildegard von Bingen, both Konrad of Megenberg and Bishop Marbodus of Rennes also wrote about them. Even the natural scientist and philosopher Paracelsus of Hohenheim, often referred to as "the patriarch of modern medicine", described, in the first half of the sixteenth century, methods of applying crystals for healing. Thus, just as there are healing plants, which have been used by those who were knowledge-able in natural healing methods from earliest times, so there are also crystals that are employed to treat physical, emotional and psychological complaints.

We now know that many of these proven therapies and invaluable knowledge were "lost" in what are called (somewhat erroneously) the Dark Ages. Nevertheless, much was also preserved and some things rediscovered – e.g. homeopathy, as promulgated by Samuel Hahnemann at the beginning of the nineteenth century.

The healing systems developed by Sebastian Kneipp in 1870, and the foundation of many schools of massage at the beginning of the nineteenth century, were of great significance for massage and physiotherapy in Europe. Their development continues right up to the present and major physiotherapy faculties all over the world have continued to make breakthroughs and establish massage as a vital part of modern medicine.

The Aurum Manus® Concept

Modern use of the term "massage" usually brings to mind ways of treating the muscles. However, this is not quite correct. If we could regard our muscles as the "workers in our bodies", it is a sad comment that they are often treated not much better than were slaves in antiquity! They are supposed to "get on with their job" and then get a "bite to eat"; and that is it. Harmonising exercises, relaxation, massage? Whatever for?

No wonder then that our muscles are often over-tense and stressed. Pain, restricted mobility, joint problems, back-

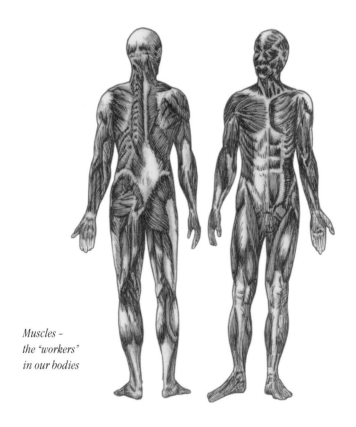

*Muscles –
the "workers"
in our bodies*

ache right through to severe headache or tinnitus are all the results – a revenge for, even – of such a negligent attitude.

What is muscular tension? How does it occur?

Our muscles produce an excess of lactic acid and its metabolic products if we constantly adopt a bad posture or are subjected to undue physical strain or demands. These products of lactic acid metabolism are transparent, gel-like substances that form in the muscles as small, solid knots over weeks and months – a condition known as myogelosis. These knots or nodules become firmly attached between the muscle fibres and, over the course of several years, may build up into mat-like layers. It is a condition that can then trigger nerve reactions and cause chronic back pain, along with many other complaints.

Relaxation through massage

Using the manual techniques of kneading, pummelling and friction (the latter from the Latin *frictio*, "to rub"), the myogeloses are broken up. Then, soon after the massage, the reduced nodules become dissolved in the blood, just like salt in warm water. This process means that any toxins deposited in these nodules are transported via the circulation to the body's filtering organ, the kidneys. For this reason, it is extremely important to drink lots of fresh water – and not carbonated beverages – in order to wash out the accumulated toxins from the kidneys. So, through this treatment and the subsequent physiological process, muscles become soft and pliable, the pain disappears, mobility is restored and one can feel much more relaxed.

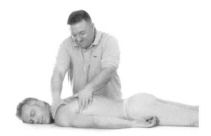

From massage to self-therapy

All of the above is merely the beginning, however. A basic requirement for its ongoing success is a general sense of inner relaxation. Furthermore, this has to be matched by an individual's decision to change his/her lifestyle. As the saying goes, where there's a will, there's a way. These changes can be based on a combination of massage, diet and nutrition, yoga and meditation – but without such an active participation, the chances for long-term improvement and alleviation of many complaints will dwindle rapidly.

Our experience of success at Aurum Manus® has been gleaned from just such a combination of massage, nutrition and yoga – and in the form of a total concept that can even be used with people who are not suffering from any complaints. Within our philosophy and treatments, the crystals used in the Aurum Manus® therapy are somewhere near the top of the list. Indeed, as there is no doubt that certain crystals have a positive effect on the body and on general health, the very same crystals employed in massage may also be worn afterwards for further beneficial effect.

The Aurum Manus®
massage purpose

The overall benefit of the Aurum Manus® massage is to create a relaxed state and regeneration of the body. At the same time, the client undergoes a kinaesthetic experience of muscular sensations as a part of the specially developed massage technique. This targeted awareness of physical experience in Aurum Manus® massage is the conscious awareness, on our part, of a holistic healing effect.

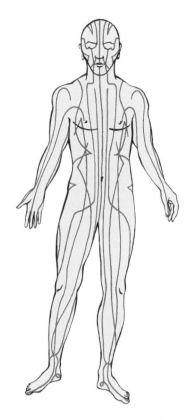

Natural energy channels of
the human body

At the same time, the massage incorporates stimulation of the energy points we have identified in the form of certain meridian and acupressure points. Crystals, such as jade, rose quartz and citrine are applied to these points after being warmed in oil, and also stimulate the vital functions of body organs. For example, jade has been found to have an extremely calming effect on the psyche as well as supporting glandular and kidney functions. As a result, the metabolism is much more able to eliminate toxins so that what traditional Indian and Chinese medicine (respectively) calls *prana* or *chi* (life energy), can flow unhindered once again. The outcome is that the body thereby regains its health, but in a gentle and natural way. After all, good things simply take a bit of time!

Warm oil massage

Warm, high-quality massage oils provide considerable support when massaging, by encouraging relaxation and also introducing their own beneficial and healing effects to the massage. Good-quality plant oils relax the skin, on which demands are also placed through the detoxification process after the massage. This is why oils produced from a petrochemical base are sheer poison; they clog up the pores in the skin and thereby cause toxins to build up. We have had very good experiences (also from an allergy angle) with sesame seed oil for the whole body and almond oil for the face. A highly controlled, organic quality of oil should be employed – this goes without saying. A crystal oil with serpentine was specially developed for Aurum Manus®, which has a relaxing and cramp-eliminating effect and also has a vitalising effect. This "Aurum Manus® massage and therapy oil" can be obtained from specialist suppliers.

The oil for an Aurum Manus® massage is warmed by means of a tea-light in the specially designed container (see illustration). A tea-light is preferable to any form of electric heating, particularly because of the crystals that are laid in the oil and warmed up there. In addition, electric warming can lead to electromagnetic pollution of the crystals and reduce their effectiveness.

Warning
Very high temperatures may be generated when warming massage oil with a tea-light in an Aurum Manus® vessel. The oil and the crystals, if not handled correctly, may lead to severe burns. Please always pay great attention to the optimal use of a temperature of 30-35 °C (about 85-95 °F).

Check the temperature of the massage oil before beginning the massage. By keeping a lit tea-light handy nearby or placing it under the oil (cup) again for a short while, the temperature can be regulated quite easily, even during the massage.

Warming massage crystals in oil

Crystal sphere massage

As a part of the Aurum Manus® therapy, we employ small crystal balls, spheres of between 3 and 5 cm (about 1 to 2 inches) in diameter. These are sometimes referred to as Chinese Balls.

Most (but not all!) are heated in massage oil as described above.

The following crystals spheres are those most frequently used when warmed.

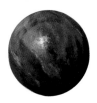

Jade or **nephrite** promotes detoxification and elimination of body toxins, and stimulates the liver, gall bladder and kidneys. They also fortify what traditional Chinese medicine calls the "kidney *chi*", our central life energy, and help with the treatment of tinnitus and migraines. They are effective here because these ailments are linked energetically to the kidney energy (tinnitus) and gall bladder (migraines). In fact, in the context of Chinese medicine and overall philosophy, jade and nephrite could be regarded as being equivalent to the *yin* and *yang* aspects of the human energy system – which is why they prove to be so effective there.

Serpentine shows a similar healing effect to jade and nephrite. Serpentine also fortifies the kidneys and stimulates efficient liver function. Thanks to its high magnesium content, serpentine also has a deeply relaxing effect and reduces stress. It has also proved to be particularly good for a facial massage. Sometimes also known as "New Jade" or "China Jade" it can be even more effective than jade or nephrite, on occasion, in reducing the symptoms of tinnitus and migraines.

Rose quartz is often described as the crystal of warm-heartedness. Emotionally, it frees the spirit while physically balancing out heart rhythms. Rose quartz also improves the circulation and enhances overall emotional sensitivity. Its most important property in massage is, however, that it creates a wonderful sense of physical well-being and a feeling of once more feeling truly at home one again in one's own body!

Citrine brings sunshine into the heart and soul. It lifts the mood, has an anti-depressive effect and encourages a long-lasting, positive attitude toward life that will survive difficulties and challenges. Citrine also helps emotional and mental "digestion" of the many daily impressions and stimuli we have to absorb – and this property is reflected physically too in that it stimulates actual digestion. Massages with citrine seem to have a harmonising effect on the nervous system and thereby on the interplay between all our internal organs.

Amethyst is the crystal of inner peace. Even in situations of worry, grief and painful losses, it helps one accept the situation and then deal with it. In conflict situations, it helps in resolution and in obtaining fair and just solutions. Physically, amethyst encourages the functions of the lungs, large intestine and skin, all of which also lead to an inner sense of purification.

The following crystals are also used in the massage as spheres, but only in a cool state (i. e. unwarmed).

Rock crystal brings about a sense of clarity, helping us to see things for what they really are. This makes it easier to avoid the illusion and the disappointment that can otherwise be the result in life. Physically, rock crystal stimulates a supply of fresh, neutral energy, which has a fortifying and rebuilding effect. Furthermore, its beneficial effect on the eyes is particularly noticeable when it is used as part of a facial massage.

Smoky quartz is the anti-stress crystal *par excellence*. It has an immediately relaxing effect – and is a particular asset in a massage if someone suffers from very severe and/or painful tensions. However, it also helps to avoid stress in everyday life, encouraging natural resilience, stamina and a more relaxed inner self.

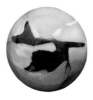

Mookaite is a crystal which "fortifies the centre" in the words of traditional Chinese medicine. It encourages inner peace and stability, but also encourages positive dynamism and enhances the energy necessary for an active life. By balancing both elements, it stimulates a full life of stimulating variety. Internally, mookaite is very beneficial for the entire stomach area and it supports/ strengthens the spleen, digestion, toxin elimination and immune system.

In practical massage applications, the small crystal spheres are guided with the hand – or just by the fingers during a facial massage. They glide over the skin easily. Their passage is lubricated by the oil being used. Only rarely is a rolling motion used, when round, tumbled stones may be employed if no spherical crystals of the desired type are available. However, small spheres are always preferable as they are much easier to handle.

Our use of these warm and cold variants is actually rather very similar way to the warm-and-cold-water treatments pioneered by Sebastian Kneipp; both utilise the energy of the warm and cold stones for healing treatments.

When massaging a client, however, it is important to identify the optimal "stimulation limits" that are appropriate both to the treatment and to the individual:

◎ not too warm or too cold!
◎ not applying the "warm" or "cold" for too long!

One's own intuition plays a part here, but *only* working strictly according to the "rules of stimulus".

The Rules of Stimulus
Weak stimulation energises ☺
Stronger stimulation supports the life energy ☻
Strong stimulation has a dampening effect ☹
The strongest stimulation is harmful ☠
✎ Note:
hold back on too much stimulation!

As described below, *four* basic massage hand movements are employed in the Aurum Manus® massage treatment.

Stroking: This movement – often also call effleurage – involves moving the hand over the skin while the shape of the hand adapts to the surface of the body. The fingers should remain closed during this movement in order to prevent rapid tiring of the hands and fingers. The stroking movement warms the skin, removes tensions and helps the muscle relax for the massage.

Kneading: The muscles are located and then pressed between the fingers and the palm of the hand, in a rhythmic, flowing movement (as with dough in bread making). This helps the initial loosening up of the muscle and then makes it more accessible to deeper treatment. The technique is sometimes referred to as deep effleurage.

Circular Pressing: Here, the muscles are pressed and pushed this way and that, in circular movements, with the little finger and the thumb. The action is sometimes called petrissage and relaxes tension over larger areas and loosens up the muscle.

Frictioning: This involves circular rubbing movements of the fingertips, knuckles or elbows (depending on the muscle involved), working deep into the muscle. This removes severe muscle tension and dissipates any myogeloses (see earlier). However, it is not a technique that should be used until the muscle has been loosened up and relaxed sufficiently using the three movements previously described.

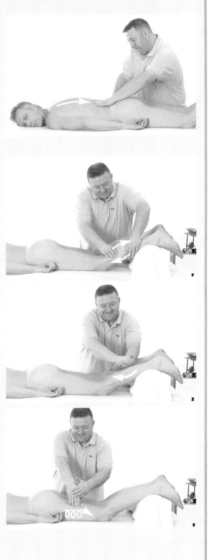

Positioning

A massage table, with a special head part, is also advantageous for the client in a prone position, so that the head does not have to be turned to the side.

Preferably, those parts not to be massaged should be covered up with a towel, and then a blanket, to maintain body temperature. The illustrations depart from this recommendation so as to present a clear view of the treatment.

If a prone position is not possible – for example, during pregnancy – the massage can also be carried out with the client lying on her side. The massage movements should then be adapted to the situation.

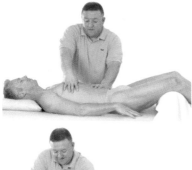

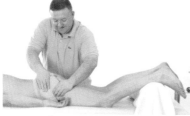

A comfortable position for the client is important

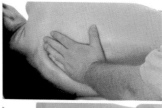

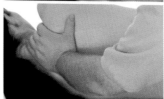

Massaging a client lying on her side

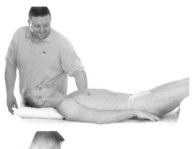

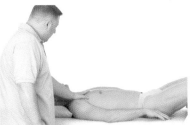

A flowing changeover (one hand always remains in contact with the body!)

A flowing motion

In order to achieve the maximum beneficial effect of the Aurum Manus® method, massage should take the form akin to that of a *continuous flow*. So, other than changing from one side of the body to the other when the client turns over, *never* remove both hands at once from the body. In other words, one hand should *always* stay in contact with the client, even when taking more massage oil for use, reaching for a crystal or moving on to the next area of the body to be treated.

In this way, a constant energy flow is maintained, which then makes the treatment a much more pleasurable experience for the client. Together with the constant replenishing of warmth by means of the massage oil and the crystal balls, this process is inherent to the distribution of relaxation in a flowing manner throughout the body – an effect that the flowing movements will deepen steadily and continuously. Its harmonising effect contributes considerably to the overall healing effect on body, mind and spirit.

The Dance of Massage

The Aurum Manus® massage is like a flowing dance between warm hands in close contact with the body of the person being massaged. In this "dance", the crystals flow in and out, as if diving in and out of a flowing stream or river. This flow enriches and revitalises every part of our being, like water filling up a vessel to the very brim.

Only massage movements that seem to be flowing like water or oil can fully benefit the client and ensure the best results. It is a picture to keep in mind throughout massage and should always remain an overall, guiding principle.

There are five basic body areas involved in our total body massage. Each has its own series of steps and the overall treatment concludes with a period of rest.

Leg massage (back)

Step 1: With the client lying prone, begin with the left leg. First, apply warm oil to moisten the whole leg, using "stroking" movements, and include the sole of the foot in this procedure. The sequence is: the calf first, then up to the thigh and back again.

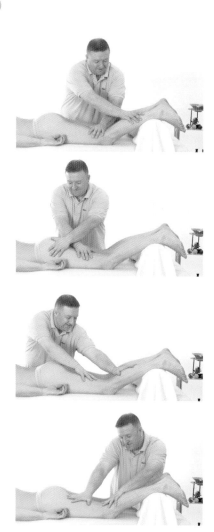

Step 2: After gently rubbing the oil over the leg, knead the calf and thigh muscles. This can be done even if the leg is bent.

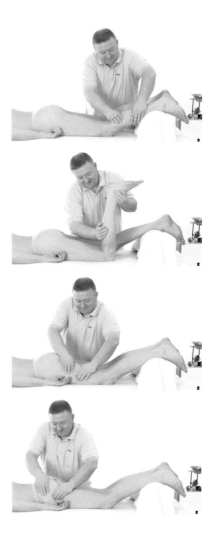

Step 3: After kneading, apply circular pressing to the muscles by means of circular movements of the little finger and the thumb.

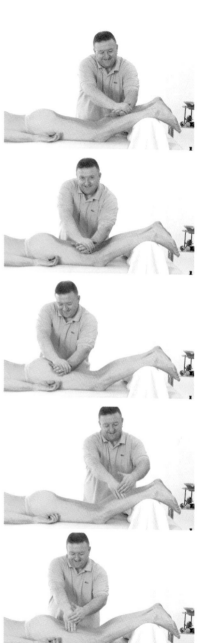

Step 4: Now move on to deep fractioning, using the fingertips. However, this stage should be undertaken with a degree of sensitivity, as the calf muscles can often be very "hardened" and tense – so if the pressure applied is too strong, it may result in more tension rather than relaxation (see the "Rules of Stimulus" above).

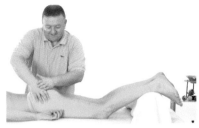

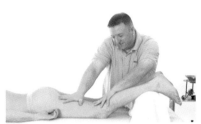

Step 5: After gentle stroking, using the flattened palms over the whole leg, switch over to the right leg. Remember: always keep one hand in contact with your client, so as not to interrupt the flow of energy!

Step 6: Continue with the same sequence of movements used when massaging the left leg.

◎ Stroking
◎ Kneading
◎ Circular pressing
◎ Frictioning

Important

The muscles are often very tensed up, so the following massage sequence should always be adhered to:

Stroking make first physical contact
Kneading loosening up the muscles
Circular Pressing intensive loosening up of muscles
Frictioning very intensive and deep work on the muscles

Never begin a massage with frictioning! However, stroking is permissible, letting it "flow in" naturally and regularly between each stage.

Step 7: After the legs have been thoroughly massaged, apply the crystals. Take one or two warmed jade or nephrite spheres from the oil cup and begin with the inside sole of the left foot. From there, and using the sphere, glide up the inside of the leg and back down along the outside. Repeat this sequence up to three times. Then carry out the same massage with the crystals on the right leg.

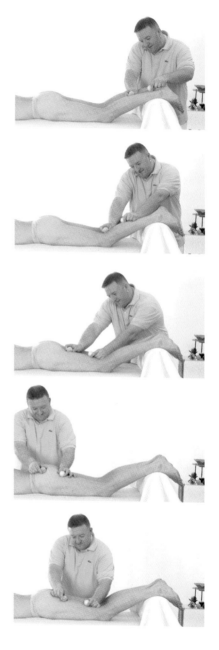

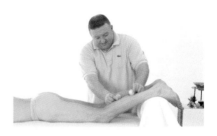

The crystals are moved with only the lightest pressure across the surface of the skin.

Afterwards, massage the legs again briefly with the palms of the hands using stroking movements and then move on to the client's back.

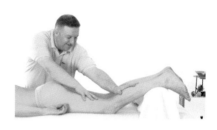

Massage time for both legs:
about 5 minutes each

Massaging the back, shoulders, neck and head

Step 1: Use lots of warmed oil to stroke the entire back, including the shoulders and neck.

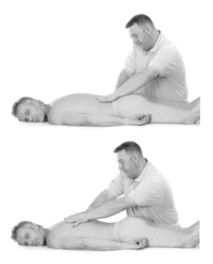

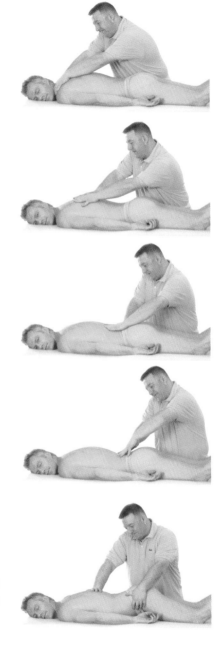

Step 2: Next, knead the top edge of the pelvis and the hips. Move up the entire flank as far as the shoulders,

on to the neck, and back down the other side, kneading all the time. In between, here too use repeated stroking movements on the back.

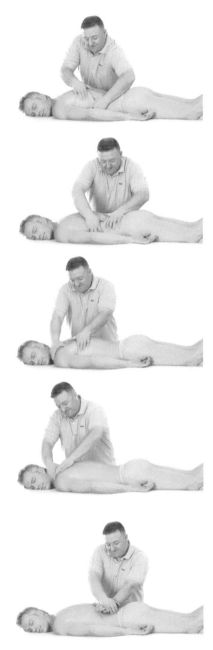

Step 3: Continue with circular pressing on the back. Using the ball of the little finger and thumb, begin at the lumbar region with medium pressure, working at

each side of the spine, and move up along the long muscles of the back to the top edge of the shoulder blade – and then back again.

Work first on the left-side muscles, then the right. Afterwards, use gentle stroking movements once again.

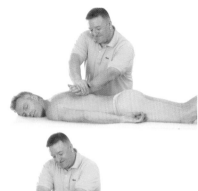

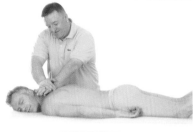

Step 4: The most intense massage movements are those used in frictioning ones, because of their in-depth effect. As with the circular pressing stage, begin at the lumbar area. Using controlled pressure of the fingertips, carry out point-like, circulatory massage along the long muscles of the back. Work first on the left muscle band, moving from lower to upper areas; then in the same way on the right muscle band. All such circulatory movements should be in an anti-clockwise direction and away from the spine.

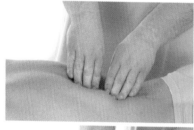

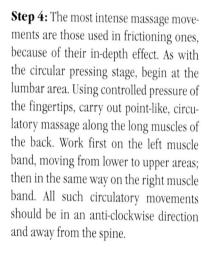

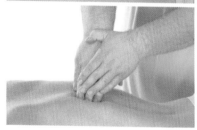

This technique is particularly helpful for work around the shoulder blades, because most tenseness is found just there. The shoulder blades should be lifted up slightly, so that they stand proud from the back. This also means that the muscles under the shoulder blades can be worked on.

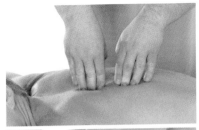

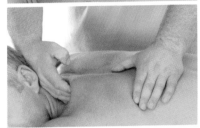

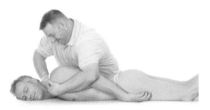

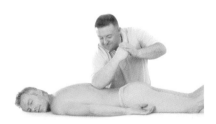

In cases of very tense muscles, frictioning can also be performed using the elbow on the long bands of back muscles.

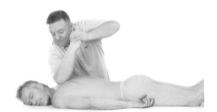

Afterwards, use two fingers to knead along the muscles, in order to loosen up any remaining tension.

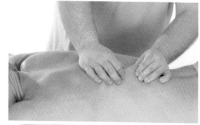

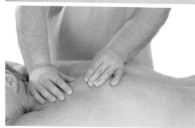

Finally, once again gently use stroking movements to massage the back.

Step 5: The next phase is the gentle pummelling and kneading of the neck muscles.

Always remember to carry out the massage very gently and slowly in the area of the neck vertebrae. Never let it become hectic or intense. Rapid or forceful movements during treatment are extremely unpleasant and disturbing for the client.

For many people it is the neck muscles that are often the most tense, yet are very sensitive. Furthermore, these tense, hardened muscles are often the trigger for headaches. For this, begin with a gentle stroking motion, then carry on with sensitive kneading movements.

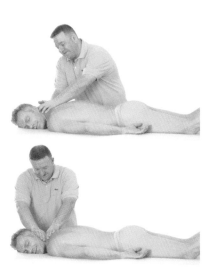

There is a whole range of pleasant and effective massage movements for the upper shoulder and neck areas. However, they should only be practised under expert supervision, ensuring at all times that the intervening (energy-removing) stroking is from the head and downwards in the direction of the loins.

Step 6: Using spread fingers push them into the hair of the client and massage the scalp with medium pressure for no more than 1–2 minutes.

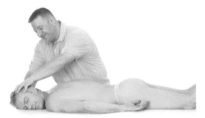

Step 7: After the above six steps, one can then use the jade or nephrite crystal balls each side of the spine in the lumbar region. The muscles on the left and the right, at the top edge of the pelvis, are plied with the warmed spheres, using stroking movements.

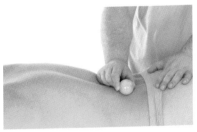

After this, the crystal ball is moved beside the spine and along the long back muscles, upwards towards the neck.

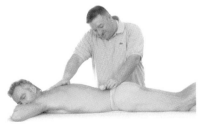

55

Using frictioning, massage the muscles around the shoulder blades (but not *on* the shoulder blades!).

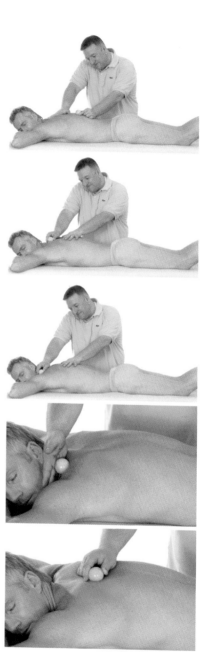

Afterwards, continue with frictioning along the long back muscles in the direction of the lumbar area. After that, use warm crystals in gentle stroking movements on the entire back.

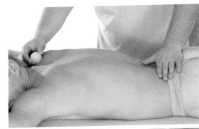

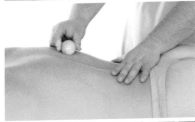

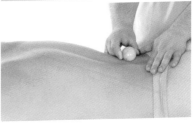

Step 8: At the end of the back massage, a cool mookaite sphere at room temperature (not warmed) is moved gently upwards over the skin, from the coccyx area and along the right-hand long back muscle. Upon reaching the top at the neck, move the crystal ball downward along the matching left-hand muscle back to where you started.

Carry this out only once. Afterwards, use stroking movements over the whole back with the flattened palms of the hands.

Massage time on the back:
approx. 20 minutes

After the above back massage, change to the other side of the body, so that the client lies on his/her back. This is the only point during the whole massage process when a small interruption becomes inevitable.

This is the immediate next phase. A facial massage comprises two parts: the initial basic massage and the crystal sphere massage.

Part 1: The basic massage

During the initial, basic massage the following rules should be observed.

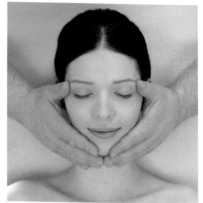

- ◎ Never massage the face vigorously.
- ◎ Always massage with soft, supple and slow movements – as if working in slow motion.
- ◎ Always massage working from below, upwards.
- ◎ Always keep at least one hand in direct body contact with the client during the massage so that the flow of energy will never be interrupted.

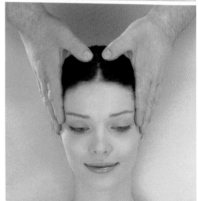

The initial massage consists of nine steps.

Step 1: At the beginning of the facial massage, both middle fingers and index fingers are laid on the front of the chin and stroking movements effected with oiled hands on the face, in the direction of the temples. Upon reaching the temples, carry out circular movements in an anti-clockwise direction.

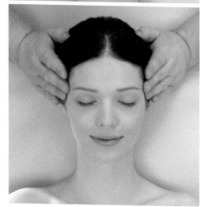

Step 2: Then place both index fingers above the top lip and stroke in the direction of the temples. Reaching the temples again, carry out the circular movements once more.

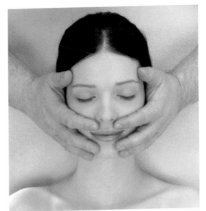

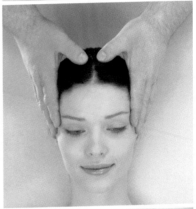

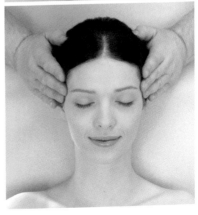

Step 3: Place the index fingers and the middle fingers underneath the eyes on the cheekbones, and stroke in the direction of the temples. Massage the temples with about 10 circular movements.

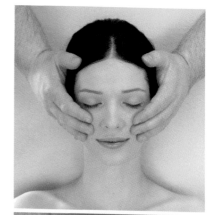

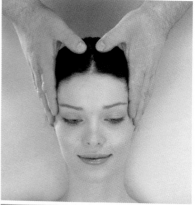

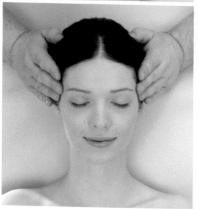

Step 4: Place the hands on the middle of the forehead and, from there, move to the temples and repeat the 10 or so circular movements on the temples.

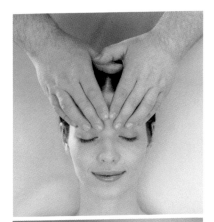

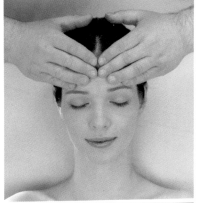

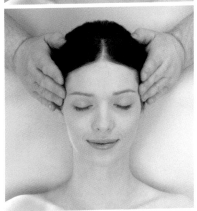

Step 5: Now gently stroke the forehead about two or three times with the flats of the hands.

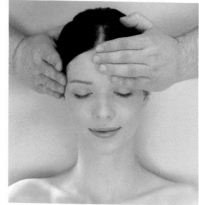

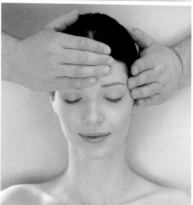

Step 6: After that, equally as gently, knead the eyebrows.

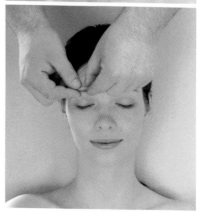

Step 7: Now stretch the neck, pulling (very) carefully. Afterwards, massage the neck and shoulder muscles.

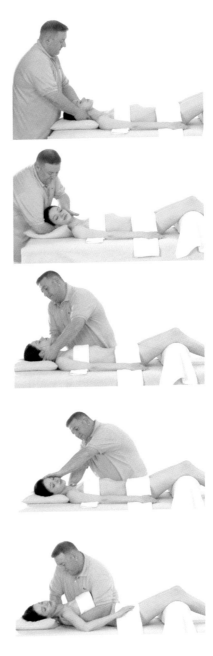

Step 8: After that, ensure that the head is again in a comfortable, quiet position. Then stroke the forehead once more.

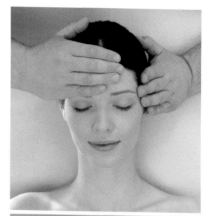

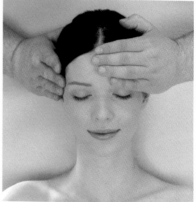

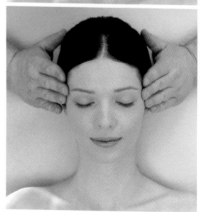

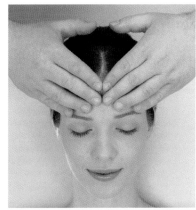

Step 9: Finally, use both index fingers and place them on the points between the inner corners of the eyes and bridge of the nose – and hold for 20 to 30 seconds. This location on the body is, in fact, the start of the bladder meridian, which regulates the relaxation of the entire body.

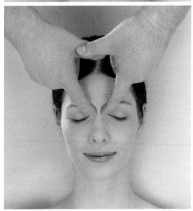

Tip

This initial basic facial massage may be varied and expanded. For example, if particular tension is evident in the jaw muscles. During an Aurum Manus® massage, special attention is paid to the muscles shown in the following illustrations.

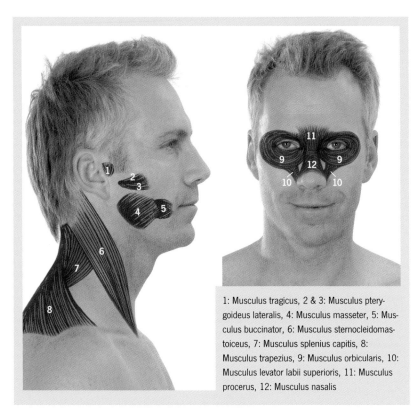

1: Musculus tragicus, 2 & 3: Musculus ptery-goideus lateralis, 4: Musculus masseter, 5: Musculus buccinator, 6: Musculus sternocleidomas-toiceus, 7: Musculus splenius capitis, 8: Musculus trapezius, 9: Musculus orbicularis, 10: Musculus levator labii superioris, 11: Musculus procerus, 12: Musculus nasalis

Important muscles in the face and neck

Part 2: Massage using small crystal spheres

This secondary facial massage consists of only six steps.

Step 1: Take a warmed jade, nephrite or serpentine ball out of the cup and place it above the bridge of the nose on the so-called "third eye" on the forehead. Allow the crystal to glide gently, without any pressure, in a clockwise direction, across the left temple to the cheekbone.

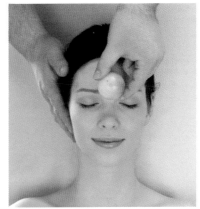

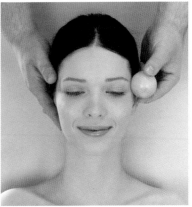

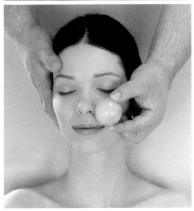

From there, move it in the direction of the ear, and from the jaw muscles to the chin.

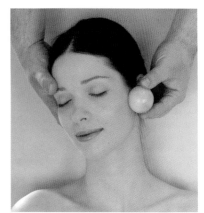

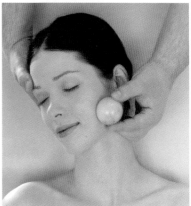

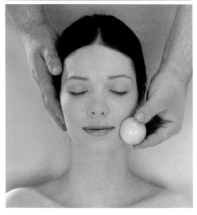

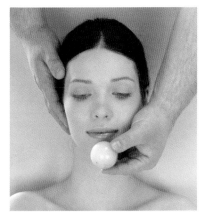

Take the crystal in the right hand and glide it on across the right half of the face, moving it towards the jaw muscles and the ear and in the direction of the cheek-bone.

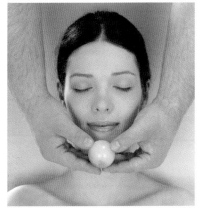

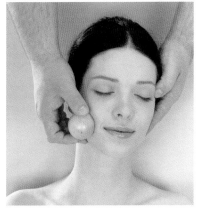

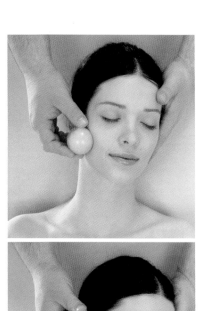

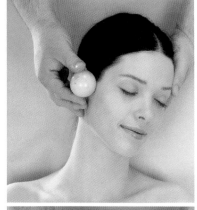

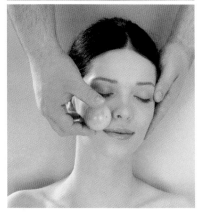

Move from the cheekbone upwards in the direction of the temple and then back to the starting point on the "third eye" on the forehead.

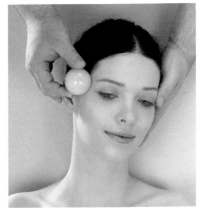

Tip
This sequence can be repeated, depending on one's intuitive feeling, with a warmed crystal of rose quartz, citrine or amethyst.

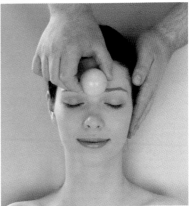

Step 2: Beginning once more at the "third eye", glide the small warmed ball of jade, nephrite, or serpentine in a clockwise direction downwards on the left side of the face. When you have reached the ear, allow the ball to "dive under" the main muscles of the back of the neck.

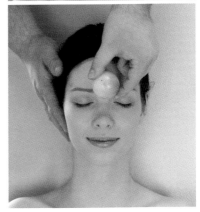

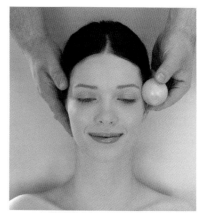

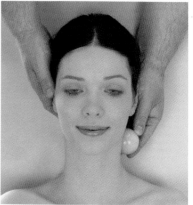

There, the neck muscles are massaged with gentle, circular movements along the hairline. The ball is moved from the left to the right hand several times, back and forth.

Warning!
Do not use the crystal ball to massage the neck vertebrae!

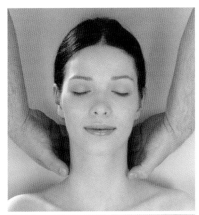

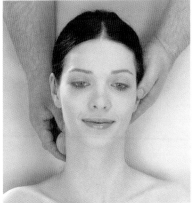

Then, holding the warm ball with the right hand, bring it down across the right half of the face, across the jaw muscles and temple and back up to the starting point in the middle of the forehead.

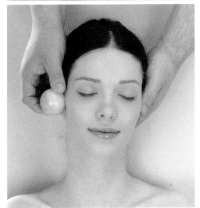

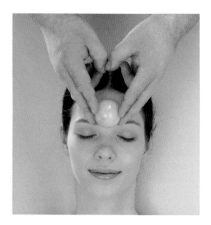

Step 3 The Full Moon: Using a warmed rose quartz crystal sphere, start once again on the forehead at the "third eye". From there, move the crystal clockwise across the left cheek and past the bottom of the lower lip, continuing high up across the right cheek, across the temple and back to the starting point of the "third eye".

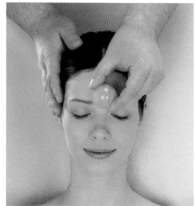

Without stopping, carry out these circular movements across the face 2 or 3 times, ending up on the forehead.

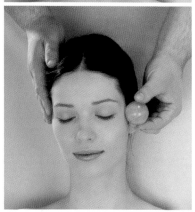

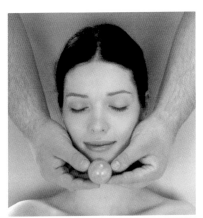

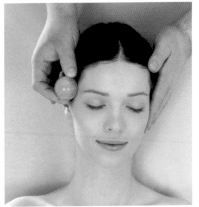

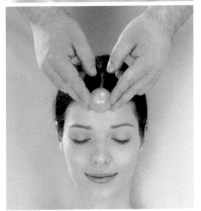

The "Full Moon" can also be carried out with just one hand and, if so desired, also using alternative spheres of serpentine, citrine and amethyst.

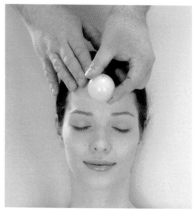

Temperature Information

The ideal temperature for working with the crystals is between 30 and 35 °C (85-95 °F. The massage movements with the crystals should be carried out in a slow and flowing manner, but never stay for too long in one spot with the crystal!

Important

Always move the massage crystals from the side where they were placed ready for use on the face, never across the face! Otherwise the oiled crystals may slip out of your hands and, depending on the height from which they fall, may cause injuries in the area of the face.

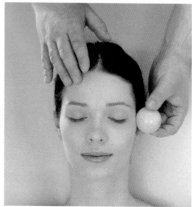

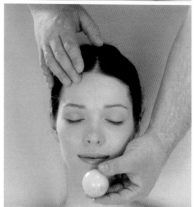

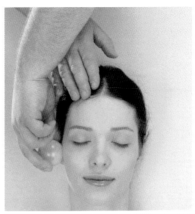

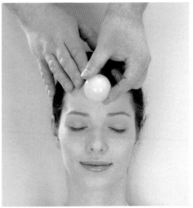

Step 4 The Spectacles: Using a cool rock crystal or smoky quartz sphere, start at the bridge of the nose and move it underneath the left eyebrow, in a clockwise direction, around the left eye and back to the bridge of the nose. From the wall of the nose, move the cool crystal ball back along the same route to the starting point between the eyes, but moving it above the eyebrow on the way back! Without stopping, glide the crystal underneath the right eyebrow, around the eye to the right-hand wall of the nose and, along the same route, back again above the eyebrow to the starting point of the bridge of the nose.

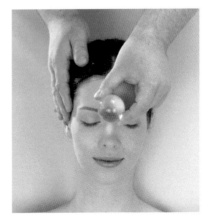

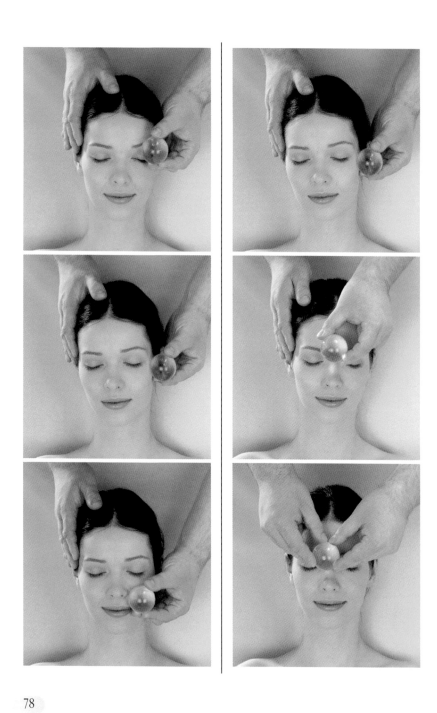

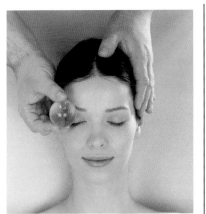

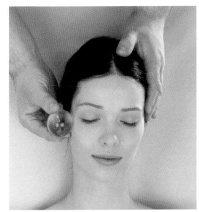

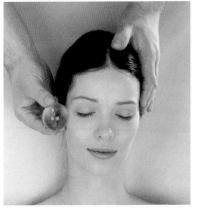

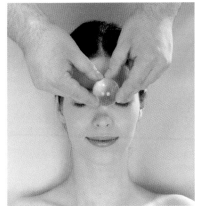

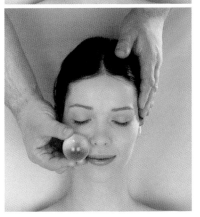

Step 5: Using the flat of the hand, gently stroke the forehead.

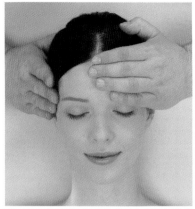

Step 6: At the end of the facial massage, lay three small cabochons (emerald, fire opal or moonstone) on the "third eye" for about 15 to 20 minutes (see illustration for the correct arrangement) and allow the client to rest for that time.

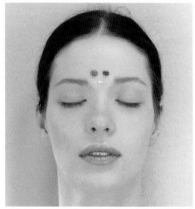

Length of facial massage:
10 minutes in total (excluding the period of rest with the crystals)

Three important energy points are stimulated and balanced with crystal treatment:

- **Green emerald** lies on the **soul point**, which also regulates the serotonin balance. Serotonin is an anti-depressive "happiness hormone".

- **Red fire opal** lies on the **mood point**, which also regulates the adrenalin balance. Adrenalin is the hormone that heightens our ability to react.

- Colourless **moonstone** lies on the **sleep point**. This point regulates the melatonin balance. Melatonin is the hormone that controls waking and sleeping rhythms.

Never begin with frictioning! Stroking, however, is acceptable as part of a natural, flowing process between the other stages.

The crystal healing treatment of these three points or centres also stimulates and balances the gall bladder meridian and the bladder meridian. Together with these two meridians, two basic abilities are balanced: the ability to approach a problem and deal with it (the gall bladder is assigned to the element wood, and is connected, among others, with the theme of "aggression") and the ability to withdraw and "let go" (the bladder meridian is assigned to the element water, and is therefore also responsible for relaxation). Balancing both these forces leads to a relaxed, trusting attitude.

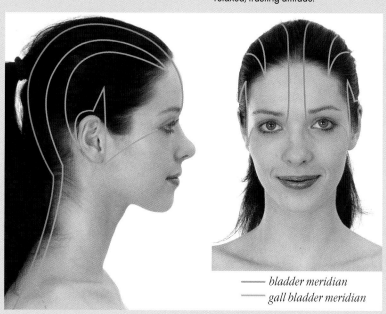

—— *bladder meridian*
—— *gall bladder meridian*

After the client has rested, make contact again gently with the right shoulder joint and massage the arms and upper body. Before starting, take more warmed oil from the oil cup and use the following five steps.

Step 1: Using the specialised grip (see illustration), hold the left arm and massage the upper arm, first with very light stroking and kneading actions, then continue with the lower arm.

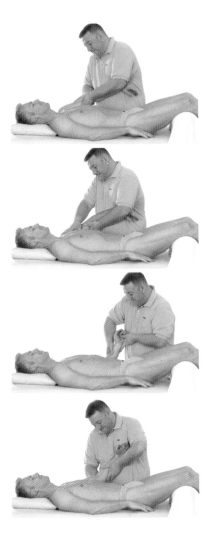

The backs of the hands should be massaged and the palms of the hands worked over firmly with the balls of the thumbs. Finally, the fingers are massaged using the so-called "corkscrew grip" (see illustration), stretching them very gently, after which the arm is stroked along its entire length, to finish off.

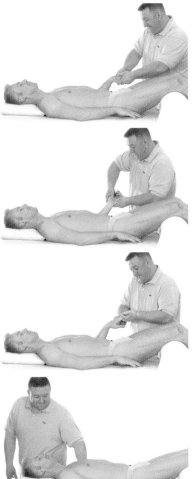

When changing over to the second arm, always ensure that the movement is conducted in a flowing motion. Begin once again with the specialised hold as in Step 1 (see illustration).

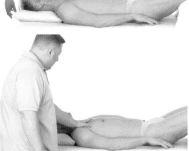

Following this, use the same movements to massage the right arm in the same way.

Length of massage for both arms: approx. 4 minutes

Step 2: Now, massage the upper body with warm oil, using gentle stroking movements.

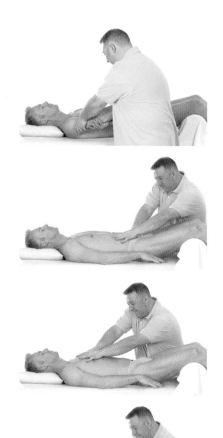

The upper chest muscles and the stomach should then be kneaded lightly.

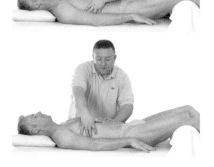

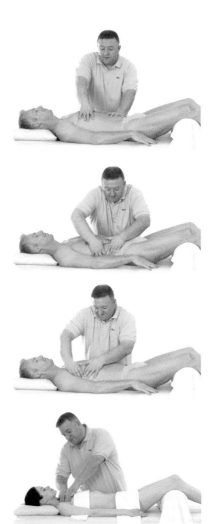

In the case of female clients, naturally, only the area above the breasts should be massaged, in addition to the stomach area.

Finally, both the chest and the stomach are massaged once more with gentle, stroking movements.

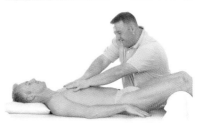

Step 3: For this step, choose between a warmed citrine, rose quartz, jade or nephrite sphere for treating the chakras (see below). Initially, the selected crystal should be placed on the throat chakra (the hollow where the larynx sits) and allowed to glide down over the heart and solar plexus to the navel and base chakra. During this movement, rest briefly at each individual chakra and carry out gentle, circular, clockwise movements.

Chakra Information

Our chakras are important energy centres that regulate the entire hormonal and metabolic activity, as well as our mental state. As chakras are control centres, treatment of them should proceed with extreme gentleness, delicacy of touch, great care and attention. In fact, it is a very delicate touch that has the greatest harmonising effect on the client.

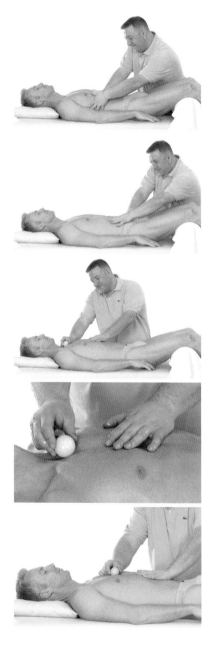

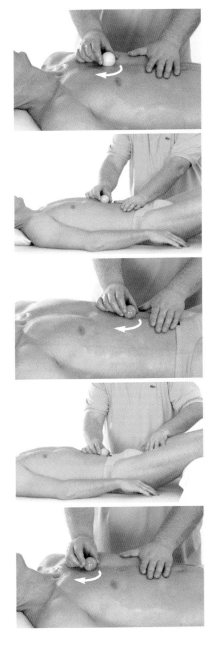

A rose quartz ball is very pleasing to use, especially for the heart chakra.

Step 4: Starting at the base chakra, above the pubic bone, use a warmed crystal sphere to stroke the abdomen gently, following the course of the large intestine (always clockwise).

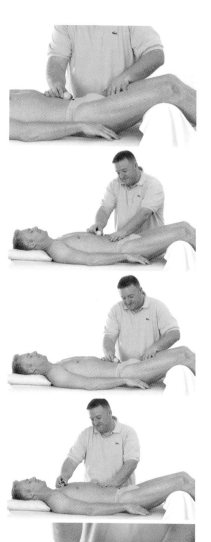

Step 5: Using a cool mookaite ball, start at the upper body with the final stroking movements. From the throat chakra (the hollow of the larynx), guide the crystal ball straight down to the base chakra (top edge of the pubic bone) and back again. This follows exactly the energy path running centrally along the body axis and connecting all the chakras on the front the body.

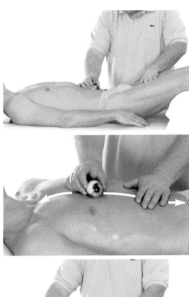

To finish with, massage the entire upper body with stroking movements using the flattened palms of the hands.

Length of massage of upper body: approx. 7 minutes

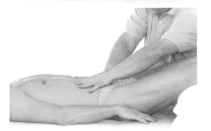

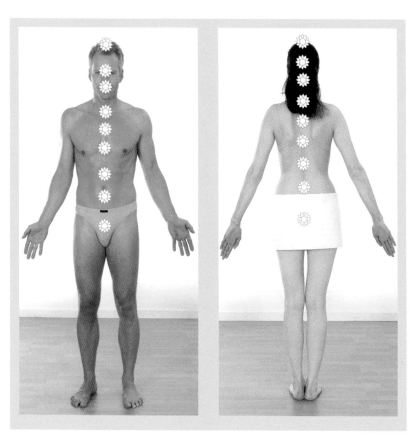

The chakras: The lowest chakra, the base chakra, is located in the area of the pubis. At the front, it opens on the level of the pubic bone, and, at the back, on the level of the transition of the sacrum/coccyx. Likewise, the crown chakra really sits on the highest point of the head. It opens at the front, at the level of the hairline (or where it ought to be) and, at the back, where many people have a twist in their hair.

The front leg massage has two main steps

Step 1: The fronts of the legs are massaged initially with gentle stroking movements, while gently rubbing on warmed oil.

Start with the left leg, stroking outwards gently, as well as kneading the thigh muscles.

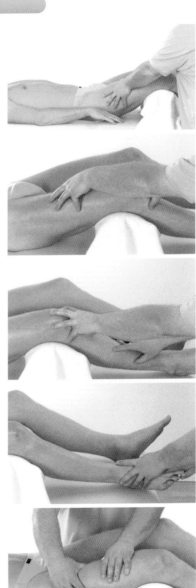

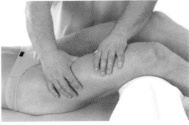

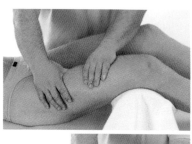

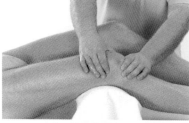

Following on, move around the kneecap and stroke the shin muscles all the way down to the feet.

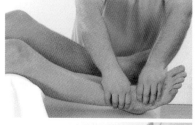

Stroke the tops of the feet and massage the soles by frictioning with the tips of the thumbs.

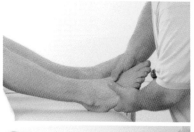

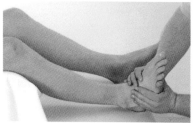

Finally, massage the legs entirely, using stroking movements.

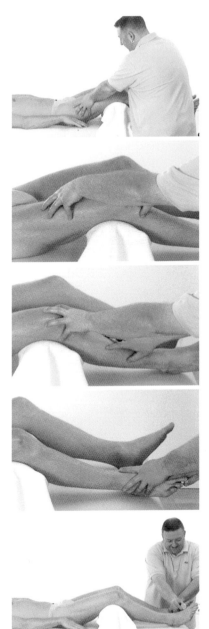

Step 2: Using a warmed jade or nephrite sphere, start with the inside of the foot. Moving along the meridian of the kidneys and liver (see illustration), guide the crystal up the inside of the leg; then change over to the outside of the leg.

Glide the crystal ball down the outside of the leg in the direction of the ankle (meridian path of the gall bladder).

Meridian Parameters

It is not important to follow the path of the meridian to the exact millimetre! The size of the sphere will, in any case, lead to contact with the meridian, thereby stimulating it.

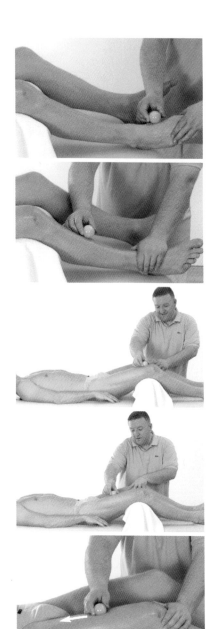

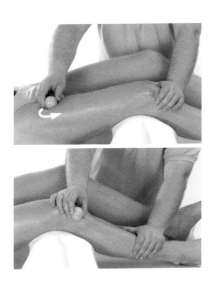

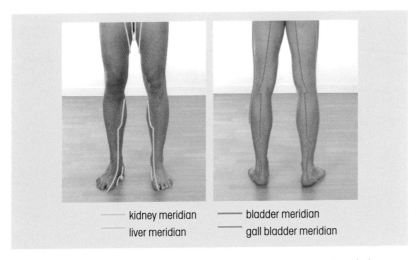

—— kidney meridian	—— bladder meridian
—— liver meridian	—— gall bladder meridian

The meridian paths of the kidneys, bladder, liver and gall bladder along the legs

⇒

This procedure can be repeated two to three times on each leg with the crystals, also circulating around the kneecaps.

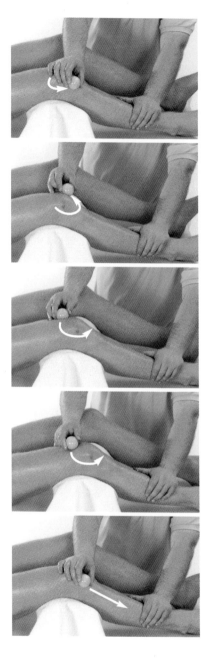

After that, also use the cool mookaite crystal ball to stroke upwards once along the inside of the leg, then down again on the outside of the leg. Afterwards, massage the leg again, using stroking movements.

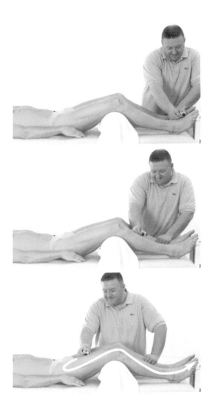

Now change over, in a flowing fashion, to the right leg and massage this in the same way.

To complete the whole massage, stroke both legs simultaneously with your hands.

Length of massage for both legs:
approx. 4 minutes each
Total massage time:
approx. 60 minutes

Rest after massage

If at all possible, after the end of the total body massage, the client should be covered warmly and then rest for a few minutes.

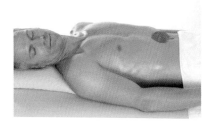

Ancillary Energising

For further energising of the body, with the client's consent, pyrites may be placed on the solar plexus chakra – but only for a few minutes, in order to avoid its sulphur component reacting with the perspiration. Orange calcite and amber are recommended for particularly sensitive people.

After the Aurum Manus® total body massage, your client should drink (at least) one glass of fresh (still, never carbonated) water. In addition, try to make a point of recommending that the client continues to drink, if possible, 2 to 3 litres of good-quality water daily in the period following the massage.

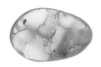

Timing of a massage

The ideal time for an Aurum Manus® massage is the late afternoon. We have observed the optimal results from treatment at this time of the day. According to the "body clock" of traditional Chinese medicine, the bladder and kidney meridians are reaching their daily peak of activity at this time. This suits the Aurum Manus® total body massage very well, as

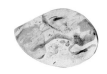

Pyrite,
orange calcite,
amber

it is geared towards treating the kidney and bladder meridians in particular (in addition to the gallbladder and liver meridians).

Ear complaints, such as tinnitus, are also connected with these meridians, usually in cases of a blockage in the liver meridian (usually stress-related) and a simultaneous problem in the kidney meridian (usually related to exhaustion).

The Aurum Manus® massage creates a balance between a build-up and a deficiency. Consequently, it is especially effective during the time of day when the kidneys are particularly active (17:00 to 19:00 hours). If this time of day is impractical, however, this need not be too much a matter of concern. It goes without saying that we feel certain that it is better to have an Aurum Manus® massage at whatever time, rather than not at all!

No matter when, the result can usually be seen, or felt...

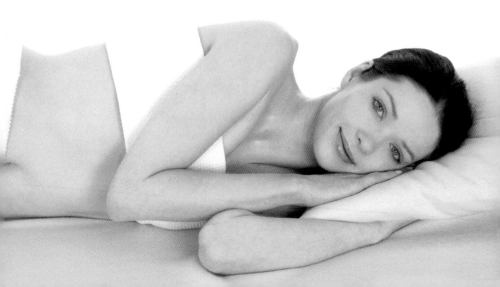

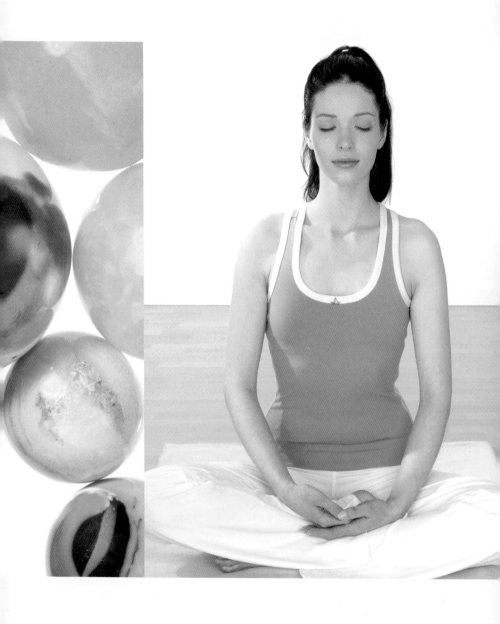

The Aurum Manus® Therapy

Man follows the Earth
The Earth follows the Heavens
The Heavens follow the Tao
The Tao follows what is
In harmony with Nature
Lao Tse, *Tao Te King*

Who Can Benefit?

◎ "I can really rely on you!", "If I didn't have you, I don't know what I'd do!" – are these things that you often hear? Additionally, what about the following statements?

◎ Do you do everything for others, for your family, friends and at work, but rarely anything for yourself?

◎ Is the thought of being "only" average an unbearable thought for you? Do you perceive your job as a daily battle for security, position, respect and success?

◎ Do you often feel as though something is driving you from within?

◎ Do you have a need for harmonious surroundings, even at the price of avoiding conflicts?

◎ Do you also find it difficult to obtain the necessary time and space to stop, rest and recharge your batteries?

Have you answered "yes" to one or more of these questions? If so, you are probably one of those people who would definitely benefit from the Aurum Manus® massage! To put it briefly, you are almost certainly making far too many demands upon yourself.

Look at it this way. Even if you are able to cope with such demands in the normal course of events, it still may well be that all that is required is the proverbial "last straw to break the camel's back". Then you will suffer the customary physical symptoms, such as headaches, migraines, tinnitus, or even loss of hearing. The breaking point may take one of many forms: for example, a change or upheaval at your place of work or in your domestic life. Even experiences which are actually positive in the overall - such as a wedding, an addition to the family, or even that well-earned annual holiday you having been looking forward to for so long - may, nevertheless, be a trigger for these or similar symptoms.

However, might there be more to these symptoms than meets the eye, especially those that appear to arise unexpectedly?

Let's take a look at this phenomenon, using the example of tinnitus. If noises in one's ears occur, it may be useful to ask whether it means that we have "had it up to here". So why are we "hearing alarm bells"? What is it in one's life that is not being heard? In his book, *Krankheit als Symbol* ("Illness as a Sign"), Rüdiger Dahlke points out that our ears, and hearing, as well as having their obvious functions, are also associated with the concept of what can best be termed "obedience". Indeed, he goes on to say that tinnitus may arise as the consequence of some inner conflict, the roots of which lie in unresolved stress. For this reason, it is not enough simply to alleviate the physical symptom (the tinnitus), but also to uncover the root of the inner emotional or psychological conflict. If this is not resolved, the symptoms will, in all probability, recur.

Much unresolved stress has its roots in feelings of fear: fear of losing one's job; fear of being abandoned by a partner; fear of failing exams; fear of not being able to cope with everyday life; fear of not being able to cope with aspects of one's own life, etc.

We sometimes use the word "angst" to describe such fears and worries. The word derives from the Latin *angus*, meaning a "narrowness" or some form of "confinement". Consequently, it is very important to determine just where and why we are experiencing such "narrowness" in our lives. For example, where is our awareness being "restricted"?

One recommended solution is meditation. This can, for example, be used to expand self-awareness and consciousness and, thereby, help to eliminate hidden fear.

In traditional Chinese medicine, a basic element assigns the emotion of fear to the element of water. Imminent, short-term fear activates the energy of the bladder meridian and triggers the "fight or flight" response. In contrast, long-term or extreme fear damages the energy of the kidney meridian.

From all of this it is apparent that unrecognised fear can lead to considerable physical problems other than just tinnitus – such as backache and spinal stiffness, hearing difficulties (even hearing loss), dizziness and headaches (including migraines).

Fortunately, we are not entirely at the mercy of such complaints. Everyone has the ability to improve his or her kidney function and inherent energy. This can be achieved by the appropriate balance between activity and rest, via a healthy diet, through the experience of true friendship, which relaxes the kidneys and assists the economical use of one's energy – and finally, of course, through Aurum Manus® massage.

How It Helps

The positive effect of the Aurum Manus® massage is based on its various components. Most obvious are the aspects and widely recognised benefits of a classic massage – where the massage movements improve the circulation in the muscles and release tension. This is supported by the use of high-grade, warm massage oils.

Meridians and chakras

Targeted stimulation of the body's natural energy channels – the so-called meridians – that form an essential part of Aurum Manus® massage encourages the

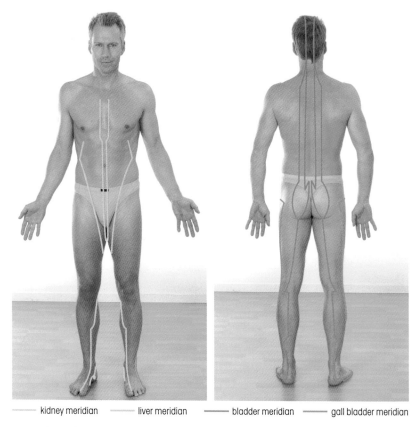

| kidney meridian | liver meridian | bladder meridian | gall bladder meridian |

Wood meridians (liver and gall bladder) and water meridians (kidneys and bladder)

elimination of absorbed waste products. In particular, it sets in motion and thereby enhances the overall detoxification process. Thus the massage concentrates very much upon on the so-called "water meridians" of the kidneys and bladder and upon the "wood meridians" of the liver and gall bladder.

These traditional Chinese elements of "water" and "wood" represent natural opposites and are equivalent to *yin* and the *yang*. "Wood" represents upwardly directed energy and "water" the downwardly directed energy. Only if/when both are in balance can the "life flow" – which constantly renews itself and regenerates the body – be maintained.

The chakras, which are familiar from the Indian/Ayurvedic tradition – and which represent another but similar way

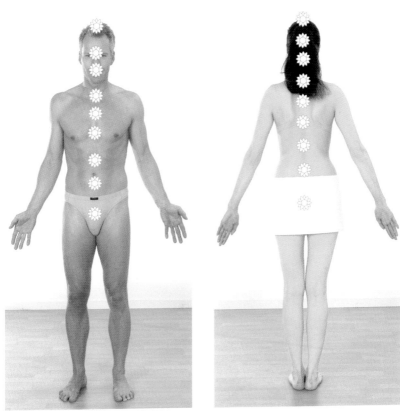

The chakras, energy centres in our bodies

of looking at energy centres within the body – are also incorporated into Aurum Manus® therapy.

There are several such points in our bodies and all our activities leave behind traces in these chakras. For example, the heart chakra was formerly also called "notched wood", in which one's conflicts have become "notched" or "embedded". Such "notches" or "scars" block the energy flow and may therefore cause one's health to deteriorate. So Aurum Manus® massage involves the chakras being activated and balanced during the course of treatment.

Crystal use

The effectiveness of the massage is further complemented and intensified by the use of small crystal spheres. Every mineral has its own unique frequency of vibration. Watchmakers have utilised this effect for decades in the production of quartz timepieces. Here, a tiny flake of rock crystal is stimulated into releasing its own frequency or oscillation at a constant rate. Time is then measured relative to this natural vibration, which is totally independent of any temperature or pressure fluctuations.

This property of crystals having their own specific frequency of vibration or oscillation because of a naturally occurring resonance within the human body,

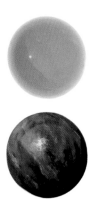

Serpentine ball (so-called "China Jade" or "New Jade") and Nephrite ball (belongs to the Jade group in the narrower sense)

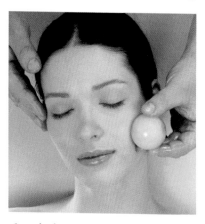

Crystal spheres used to "dissolve" blockages

means that they are capable of removing any "blockages" and reactivating damaged or affected functions of the body.

The inherent vibrations of the mineral jade, in particular, have an especially strong effect on the kidney and bladder meridians, and this is something that we make use of in Aurum Manus® massage. It is a property of jade that has been known by Chinese doctors for hundreds of years and is the reason why it is regarded as sacred in China, where it represents the balancing of opposites and the harmony between *yin* and *yang*.

From a mineralogical point of view, "jade" is also a generic term for the associated minerals called jadeite and nephrite, which also owe their names to their healing powers. Etymologically, the word jade derives from the Spanish *pietra de ijada*, which means "loin stone". Nephrite comes from the Latin *lapis nephriticus*, which means "kidney stone" (in turn form the Greek *nephron*, " kidney").

In China, serpentine is also included as part of the jade group of minerals as it is largely found in the same geological

106

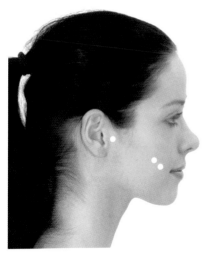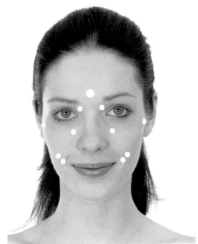

locations, has a similar physical appearance and is also an effective healing crystal for the kidneys.

In addition to jade, other crystals, such as amethyst, rock crystal, citrine, mookaite, smoky quartz and rose quartz, are also employed in Aurum Manus® massages.

When carrying out specific treatment for headaches or tinnitus, Aurum Manus® therapy follows up the facial massage with stimulation of facial energy centres using a laser-acupuncture device.

This has proved to be a highly effective and energy-enhancing way to round off the treatment.

Additional Benefits

Combating Stress

Aurum Manus® therapy has further benefits that arise from its overall ethos of being what might be termed a "stress buster". In fact, the lasting and success of the Aurum Manus® therapy is based, first and foremost, upon dealing with and eliminating underlying stress. But what is stress – and how does it arise?

The nature of stress

Stress has been defined as "an intense self-demand for achievement" or as "heightened anxiety, pressure or emotional strain". In fact, "stress" is really an abbreviated form of the word "distress". With its associations of mental pain and anguish this is a word that describes very aptly the entire phenomenon of stress –

something that puts us under pressure, causes internal tension and which may indeed lead to mental pain and anguish.

We all have to deal with a certain amount of stress in our lives, but the limits of tolerance vary considerably. The stress level that may be stimulating for one person may be a real burden for someone else. Stress makes sense if a certain goal is to be attained. Adrenalin is the "achievement" hormone and is produced to a lesser or greater degree, depending on the intensity of the pressure. For example, it is essential if one requires a sudden "spurt" for a limited period of achievement and activity. However, if it is produced when one is in a perpetual rush or feels under constant pressure there appears to be no "safety valve" and it can cause health problems. This is the stage when stress can have a negative effect on the body, the immune system will react adversely and the nerves will suffer. Therefore, it is important to recognise the point at which stress is no longer tolerable and turns into true emotional and mental pain.

Stress and the body

Then there is also the question of what is actually going on inside us during times of stress. Because stress levels are particularly critical factors in overall levels of health, their combination with other factors - such as cigarette smoke (including passive smoking), over-indulgence in drinking coffee or alcohol, consumption of artificial colouring agents, preservatives and synthetic sweeteners, nitrite and nitrate residues in foods and in certain medications - is extremely important. These are all substances and compounds that remove vitamins and minerals from the body, which we all need for a healthily functioning immune system. If one is subject to stress-related output levels of adrenalin without any accompanying physical activity (e.g. sport, gym use and so forth), too many

Our nerves are taxed by constant stress, which, in turn, affects the whole body, as well as the mind and the spirit.

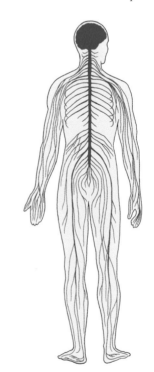

free radicals are created within the body. These free radicals occur especially in incompletely burned oxygen molecules which, in turn, trigger oxidation processes in the body's cells. The fatty substances that occur naturally in these cells then become "rancid"; they form plaques, consisting of fine layers of fats, which are deposited on the walls of the vessels, thereby raising blood pressure.

In summary, stress, together with other adverse factors, creates a physiological situation that may accelerate a tendency to damage and to illness. In the long term, both the immune system and thus the production of antibodies, is compromised. A large number of chronic diseases may arise; for example, arterial heart disease, severe headaches, allergies and tinnitus. The kidneys, which have a filtering and metabolic function in the body, are hardly able to cope with the excessive amount of toxins. This, in turn, causes severe metabolic disturbances.

These metabolic disturbances will also have a negative effect on the ability of the meridians, which are the energy channels of our bodies, to conduct energy. Humans have a widely branching network of these 'supply lines', which supply all the cells and organs with energy (prana or chi). To put it simply,

The blood vessels are also detrimentally affected in the long term

No life without a meridian system

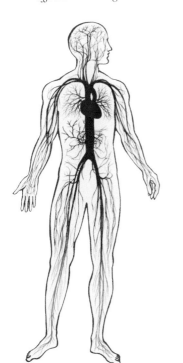

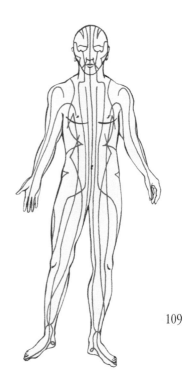

everyone has their own electrical circuit in their body. Without this energy, there would be no life!

Dehydration is another associated harmful condition in this context. There is a very real danger of the body "drying out" if we are often so absorbed in our work that we simply forget to take drinks. It is vital to drink plenty of pure, still (non-fizzy/uncarbonated) water of low mineral content or to take various kinds of green and herbal tea (no black tea!). Other drinks and proprietary beverages that have added sugar or artificial sweeteners (aspartame, etc.), and even an excess of coffee, will tend to leach water and essential minerals from the body. In contrast, water will wash out toxins deposited in the kidneys and serves as the agent for transporting minerals around the body. If a person is dehydrated, energy flow in the body becomes inadequate and the kidney meridians, being associated with the element of "water" are particularly affected. Note that the kidney meridians are also involved in the energy supply to the ears - hence the connection with tinnitus.

Recognising stress
The general effects of stress can be identified by one's behaviour, through physical signs and in emotional reactions.

Behavioural aspects:
- sudden attacks of needing to eat excessively ("frustration eating")
- smoking excessively
- impulsive behaviour that is out of character
- constant restlessness
- inability to relax
- sleep disturbance
- communication problems with colleagues or at home

Physical aspects:
- pains unconnected with muscles
- back pain
- tension in the neck
- headaches
- nausea

Emotional aspects:
- constant stress may wear one down emotionally in the long term
- constant tiredness
- mental lethargy
- lack of interest in everyday things
- problems in concentrating
- self-doubt

Overcoming stress
As we have seen, stress is a very complex business. It can only be overcome on deeper, permanent levels by a combination of measures.

Naturally, in the long term, such measures are aimed at life changes. Yet, until

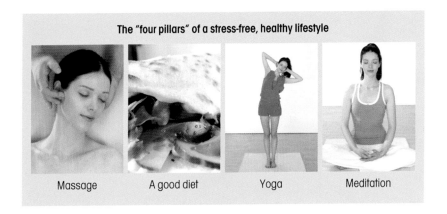

The "four pillars" of a stress-free, healthy lifestyle

| Massage | A good diet | Yoga | Meditation |

these changes can be brought about – and providing that the change itself does not, ironically, become an additional stress factor in itself – the first step is to engage in treatments or activities that will provide relief and release. Among these are massage, physical exercises, relaxation, sufficient sleep, detoxification and a good diet.

Step by step, this will lead to what one can call the "four pillars of a good lifestyle" – massage, nutrition, yoga and meditation – long recognised in Far Eastern philosophies and practised successfully in Asia for a long time. Many people following such lifestyles and belief systems manage to live with visibly less stress and also longer than those in modern, Westernised cultures and societies – and do so in spite of considerable difficulties. It is something to make one think!

Aurum Manus® therapy believes these "four pillars" are the key to good health and long-term prevention of stress and its accompanying effects. Thus, in the following sections, we will consider these principles in the way in which they are an integral component of Aurum Manus® therapy.

Complementary Exercises

Having already described in detail the Aurum Manus® massage in the first and second parts of this book, this is the point to consider what can be done if massage is unavailable, impractical or you are between massage sessions. In all cases, the aim is to support and maintain the effects of the massage and its principles – so that the following physical exercises, like the massage, specifically activate and strengthen the "water" and "wood" meridians.

For kidneys and bladder

Stand upright, with the feet parallel (without forcing the knee joints backwards!) and stretch your arms upwards.

Next, stand on tiptoe and walk forward a few steps – and then back again. Now place the whole foot on the floor again (without pressing the knee joints backwards!) and bend the upper body downwards with outstretched arms as far as possible. Breathe out throughout this movement.

Now, bend forward, until the fingertips (if possible) touch the floor. Breathe deeply "into" this stretch.

Now straighten up again slowly, from the downward position upwards, "vertebra by vertebra". Again, breathe out during this movement.

Now, when you have straightened up completely again, try to sense the beneficial energy flow in your back and legs.

Afterwards, sit on the floor and stretch your legs out and apart as far as possible. At the same time, stretch out your arms.

Now, bend forwards, keeping your back as straight as possible (but without trying to stay so stiff that you feel cramped!), until you can take hold of your legs or feet. You should breathe out while doing this movement. While breathing out slowly, you can add a little more to the forward bend with each extra amount of air exhaled. While doing this, feel the breathing movement in your pelvis.

Now straighten up again while breathing in and move your legs together again. Again, feel that very agreeable flow of energy afterwards.

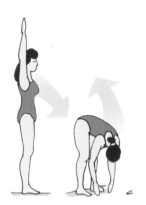

Exercise 1 for the kidneys and the bladder

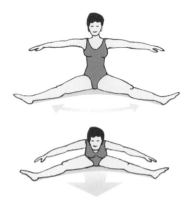

Exercise 2 for kidneys and bladder

For liver and gall bladder

Kneel on the floor and place your feet in such a way that you are touching the floor with your knees and toes.

Then bend back, while breathing out, and alternately touch the left and right ankle with one hand. Repeat with the other hand.

Then, when breathing out again, allow yourself to sink further backwards, so that you can support yourself with both hands on your ankles. Breathe deeply into this stretch and into the line of the meridian.

Retain this position for a while. Then, while breathing out, straighten up again and, for a moment, allow yourself to feel the energy flow in your legs, stomach and chest.

Now, while keeping your shoulders in contact with the floor, allow the knees to sink to the right on an out-breath, until they are lying flat on the floor. Now breathe into this twist of the spine, so that your back is relaxed. When breathing in, raise the knees up again and then, on an out-breath, allow the knees to sink to the left-hand side. Again, breathe into this stretch.

Finally, straighten the knees up again on an out-breath and stretch out your legs. Feel the flow of energy in your back and sides.

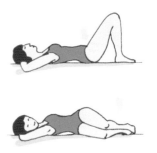

Exercise 2 for the liver and gall bladder

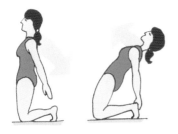

Exercise 1 for the liver and gall bladder

Afterwards, lie on your back and fold your hands behind the back of your neck. Breathing out, place your legs, bent at the knees, so that your feet and legs are close together.

Breathing out with every movement is very important, as it encourages relaxation and helps the stretch. If you carry out the movements when breathing in, or even hold your breath, you will merely have the opposite effect of creating tension and blocking the meridians. For this reason, pay particular attention to your breathing and carry out all movements of these exercises consistently while breathing out.

Also allow gravity to work with those movements that include bending and sinking down. Do not push with your muscles, but instead allow the movement to flow with a relaxing motion.

When carried out correctly, these exercises will improve the energy flow in the meridians and in the kidneys, bladder, liver and gall bladder. Simultaneously, they have a relaxing effect while stimulating detoxification and the metabolism. You should, therefore, drink plenty of fluids after carrying out these exercises. Their overall effect will be heightened by regular repetition, taking up only a few minutes every day, but being well worth the effort!

Relaxation and Sleep

A further aspect of relaxation is having a sufficient amount of healthy sleep. Those who are under a lot of pressure during the day especially require relaxation through sleep. The energies of the kidneys, bladder, gall bladder and the liver meridians are all regenerated during rest at night. This is amply demonstrated by such experiences as, say, an increase in backache at the end of the day, but which disappears like magic after eight hours of sleep. This relief is a direct result of the bladder meridian being replenished with energy overnight.

Disturbed and interrupted sleep patterns are problems particularly cited by people who are under a lot of stress. For some, it is thoughts from the day that will not go away, which go around and around and do not allow any rest. Others find that they cannot get to sleep because of persistent noises in their ears. Yet others find they can drop off to sleep, but then wake up at some time in the middle of the night, lying awake for hours without being able to get back to sleep. Sometimes the only way out seems to be to resort to sleeping tablets - the only problem being that such medication simply exacerbates the problem in the long run.

The best way to get to the root of a sleep problem is by taking specific, recommended measures, including always going to bed at the same time (every day, even at weekends) in order to achieve a

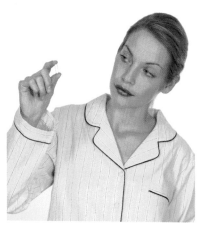

Sleeping tablets cannot provide "good sleep"

"training effect". In fact, the Aurum Manus® therapy advises not watching television before going to bed!

Instead, it is much better to take a short walk before bed; 30 minutes out is quite sufficient. Maybe a walk "around the block", perhaps with your partner, could become a beneficial habit. If you still want to read for a while in bed, please do so; but nothing exciting (no "whodunnits" or thrillers!) or to do with work. If you can't immediately get to sleep, do not toss around in bed for hours on end. Better to get up, have a hot drink (drinking alcohol *is not* a sleeping aid) and then lie down again.

An additional and valuable means of relaxing is learning a suitable relaxation technique – such as autogenic training, progressive muscle relaxation á la Jacobson, or the Feldenkrais method. Traditional routines like Qi-Gong, Tai Chi or yoga, which all combine relaxation with healthy movement, are also highly recommended. These days, they can be learned in courses almost everywhere.

Finally, in cases where disturbed sleep cannot be eliminated despite all manner of measures being taken, it is worth looking at the possibility that there may be negative, disruptive or detrimental sources in the vicinity of the bed itself, or within the space in which one sleeps. It may sound rather strange, but why not consider having the bedroom checked out by a dowser or inspected for biological and structural problems (e.g. building materials and things like moulds, fungus, mites, etc.). After all, we spend a good third of our lives in the bed, and this third should definitely be relaxing!

Detoxification

The Aurum Manus® massage promotes detoxification and waste elimination. Removal of such absorbed toxins from the body is dependent on a good supply of sufficient fluids otherwise they will become lodged at some other location within the body. This is why one of the foremost post-massage acts – and at any other time – is to drink two to three litres of clean, fresh water daily.

It cannot be repeated often enough that the beverages one chooses play an

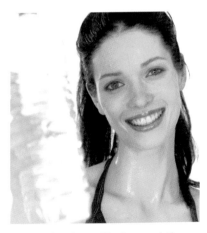

Two to three litres of fresh water daily are the body's minimum requirement!

115

important part. Preference should always be given to good, non-fizzy (uncarbonated) water. But various teas (herbal teas, fruit teas, green tea) and highly diluted fruit juices may also be taken. Sweetened or caffeine-containing fizzy drinks (even if they contain "only" artificial sweeteners, rather than sugar), coffee and black tea, as well as milk (although the latter is counted as a food rather than a drink) are far less suitable.

However, we do not detoxify our bodies through the kidneys alone. The process also takes place via the intestines. This is why a regular bowel function and healthy "flora" in the intestines are particularly important. The quality of digestion and of elimination, as well as the ability of the immune system to function properly, all depend upon a healthy intestinal flora. Feelings of being overfull, bloated and having wind, constipation or diarrhoea, reactions to certain foods, allergies and eczema may all point to a disturbance in the intestinal process. The restoration of a normal physiological intestinal flora is the goal of targeted intestine symbiosis treatment, which can be carried out by either a doctor trained in naturopathy or by an alternative practitioner.

Acid-alkaline Balance

Many of the metabolic processes in our bodies produce acids, which have then to be counteracted (neutralised) by alkalis, in order for the pH level of the body to remain stable around the point of chemical neutrality. The pH value is a chemical scale of measurement that provides an indication of acidity and alkalinity. It ranges from the value pH 1 for total acidity, to pH 14 for total alkalinity. Therefore a neutral solution or liquid, such as pure water, has a pH value of 7. Similarly, blood ought to remain more or less neutral, ideally having only a very narrow range between pH 7.3 and pH 7.4 (technically, this is ever so slightly alkaline, in fact) and it should be maintained at this level if there are to be no fundamental health problems. A number of natural "buffer systems" are in place to ensure that this chemical balance is maintained. Firstly, there are the lungs, which remove carbonic acid in the form of breathing out carbon dioxide. Then there are the kidneys, which eliminate acid as a constituent of urine, but for which sufficient fluid has to be available. The intestines, too, are involved in the de-acidification of the body. Thereafter, if there is no other way, even the mucous membranes and the skin are used as "emergency exits" (although this process, in turn, tends to create a susceptibility to colds and skin problems).

Any remaining acids that cannot be eliminated through these normal routes – the lungs, kidneys, intestines, mucous membranes and skin – are instead combined by the body with neutralising minerals (especially calcium-based compounds) and are then deposited in the connective tissues. This creates waste substances, which, in turn, may result in a lack of calcium for other functions in the body. For example, it has now been established that there are children already showing signs of osteoporosis (brittle bones) because of calcium deficiency. This is due to over-acidification, the root of which is all too often the excessive consumption of lemonades and other soft drinks containing sugar and carbonic acid – this latter being carbon dioxide dissolved under pressure in the liquid of the drinks in order to produce their characteristic fizziness.

The pH factor of urine can be tested with a simple indicator strip available from a pharmacy. As explained above, a pH value of 7 is neutral, which means acids and alkalines are evenly balanced, with anything below 7 being acidic and those above 7 being alkaline. It is not enough simply to check the pH value on a daily basis, as there may be fluctuations throughout the day. As a rule, urine is acidic in the morning because of the increased amounts of acid excreted during the night. In contrast, after meals, there should be a definite alkaline value.

Among other things, the pH value can be influenced by our diets. Some foods cause an increase in acid-formation, while others cause a shift into the alkaline range.

Among those that create acids are proteins (especially animal proteins), carbohydrates (such as sugar and products made of white flour). However, consumption of alcohol, coffee and nicotine also add to the acidification process.

On the other hand, foods that create an alkaline climate include most vegetables, fruits and nuts, as well as naturally occurring fats and oils. The process of de-acidification can be boosted by consumption of such foods, preferably combined with the mineral metallic elements potassium, magnesium and calcium.

Bathing (complete or partial baths, for example in the form of a footbath) with a bath salt of an alkaline-mineral base encourages the process of acid elimination through our organ with the greatest surface area – our skin. If there is no time or opportunity for a bath, kidney or liver poultices containing alkaline-mineral bath additives may also help detoxify the body.

A Healthy Diet

From the above consideration of the acid–alkaline balance required of the body, it must be obvious that diet has a great influence on our sense of well-being and health. In this context, it ought also to be clear why the Aurum Manus® therapy also places great importance on diet.

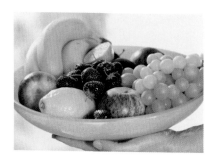

An avowed goal should be to eat foods which have a high content of vitamins, minerals and trace elements, but as little as possible of animal proteins and fats. Carbohydrates should consist mainly of those in fruits, vegetables and salads, pulses and wholegrain cereals. In particular, their content of vitamins B1 (thiamine), B2 (riboflavin), B6 (pyridoxine), B12 (cyanocobalamin), C and E, as well as magnesium, selenium and zinc should determine the choice of foods. Tiredness, lethargy, lack of concentration, sleeping disorders, heightened susceptibility to infections or heart and circulatory problems may all indicate a lack or deficiency of these.

Special attention should be paid to the so-called antioxidants, among which are vitamin C, vitamin E and secondary plant substances. They are able to render free radicals harmless, the latter being substances which are increasingly produced in the body in situations of stress and which may lead to damage to your health.

In most cases, one can obtain a suffi-cient supply of these important substances through a diet containing a high proportion of fresh food – including raw fruits and vegetables – as well as a balanced level of carbohydrates, protein and fats. In other words, fruit, vegetables, wholegrain cereals, organic (or brown) rice, pulses, nuts, milk products and cold-pressed oils really do belong on our daily diet sheet.

All meals should be prepared with ingredients that are as fresh as possible. Furthermore, wherever and whenever possible, they should be consumed in a peaceful atmosphere. Only in this way can we supply our bodies with what they require for maintaining our health.

Products made with white flour, sugar, artificial sweeteners, margarine and hard fats, along with the frequent consumption of meat (including cold meats and sausages, which contain phosphates) may be detrimental to your health.

Finally, if any uncertainty about a good daily diet remains, individual advice on nutrition may be of help. Ask your doctor or alternative practitioner, who should be only too pleased to give you support in this undertaking.

Prevention – Philosophy and Practice

For just about everyone, prevention of many ailments and conditions really begins with their parents during the months of pregnancy. Ideally, any parents-to-be should first get rid of their own health deficits and harmful indulgences, avoiding especially food that is poor in vitamins (such as "fast food"), along with sweets, confectionery, alcohol, cigarettes and social drugs, in order to avoid passing them on to their children during the early years of their lives.

A normal newborn human being usually arrives in this world in a perfect state of health. From then on, it is important to maintain this condition and to take responsibility for the growing child. After all, the first role models for all children are their parents - be they blood relatives or by early adoption - and according to the saying "The apple does not fall far from the tree".

Some kindergartens in Asia teach children foot reflexology massage from an early age, and in later years instruct them in yoga or Tai Chi for their physical well-being. This is often accompanied by lessons in meditation as a way of expanding the child's consciousness and spiritual well-being. Wherever social circumstances permit, a good, balanced and natural diet completes this picture of care and forms a total health concept, which many in the West often only know about from books. This very old Eastern concept of good health consisting of the previously explained "four pillars" of a balanced diet, exercise, massage and meditation, is the basis for a long, healthy life.

In developed, Westernised industrial society, along with our accelerating "progress" and affluence also came the modern "civilisation" diseases such as stress, deadline pressure and existential angst. Added to these can be other burdens such as our increasing environmental concerns, while pollutants in our food contribute to the harmful effects on our health. It is thus our own responsibility to ensure that all that is harmful is kept away from our bodies.

Therefore, in order to prevent illnesses, one must first need to understand how they arise. This the help that the third part of this book is intended to provide. Yes, there really are ways of changing things - and it is never to late to start!

In the end, it is only active cooperation that can provide the foundation for any kind of healing and the success of all treatment and lifestyle concepts. Without this cooperation, the outlook for improvement diminishes considerably.

A lifestyle change, which is all-inclusive and everyday in its application, based on diet, exercise and relaxation, in association with the Aurum Manus® massage, is one that contains undreamed-of possibilities!

119

Yoga

Yoga can also be an enormous help for the encouragement of physical and spiritual health. But what is yoga?

Some people think that it is like meditation; others see it merely as a form of physical exercise. In reality, yoga is a collective term and contains two aspects: a physical one and a spiritual one. In the West, it is physical yoga (called hatha yoga) with which most are familiar. Many courses are available and at many levels, where people of any age, for various different reasons, come together to learn and practise it.

Hatha yoga is a natural, physical/spiritual holistic method of physical exercise that produces an intense effect on a deeper, spiritual level. The postures, called asanas, train both the entire internal and external muscles of the body, strengthen the back and assist in the prevention of all kinds of human "wear and tear" and associated symptoms. By carrying out breathing, concentration and relaxation exercises, the person practising yoga experiences inner peace and calm, while physical tensions caused by a hectic pace of life, with its excessive demands and stress, are dissipated.

Many people who practise yoga sleep better, experience mental refreshment, enjoy increased vitality and happiness in their daily lives and experience a greater awareness in carrying out even the most mundane of daily tasks. Yoga postures have a positive effect on heart function, circulation, digestion and elimination of toxins, etc. It works this way because its inherent discipline of exercises and concentration on a single thing are carried over to other areas of life.

The actual word "yoga" derives from ancient Sanskrit, meaning "union of body, spirit and soul". Indeed, hatha yoga is a particularly good basis for following the spiritual path of yoga – for example, for concentration and the correct sitting posture for meditation.

However, there are also many seekers after a deeper meaning to life, who do not practise physical yoga but but have turned directly to its meditation aspects. Here, within yoga, there are three basic questions that have occupied human thought, philosophy and religion from the very beginning.

◎ Where do I come from?
◎ Who am I?
◎ Where am I going?

Today, there are many people seeking a new consciousness for their inner self-expression and awareness who are also involved with these and similar central questions. They realise that the body is not "everything". Rather, it can provide the means and opportunity and become a departure point from which to develop and evolve – physically, intellectually and also spiritually. In many instances, such seekers have also sought the help of a competent, spiritual teacher.

To introduce you, as the reader, to yoga, here is an initial, short sequence of exercises that are simple to carry out and which, with regular practice, will lead to a noticeable clearing of the mind, body and spirit. Should you wish to become more deeply involved in yoga, it ought to be relatively easy these days to find courses and teachers locally and at the required level and duration.

A modest programme
Stand up straight, with your feet parallel (without pushing the knee joints backwards!) and stretch out your arms horizontally to the sides. Breathe a few times quietly in order to relax.

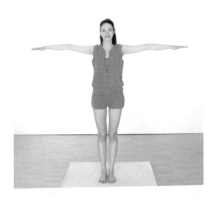

Then, with your arms held horizontally, twist to the right around your own axis, as far as you can without using pressure or force. Remain briefly in this position and breathe quietly to relax. When breathing out, you may be able to extend the twist a little by a few centimetres.

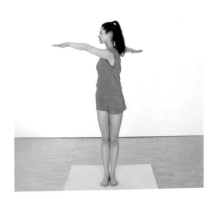

Return to the initial position.

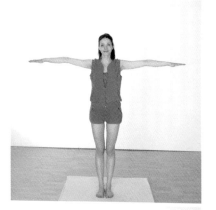

Now repeat the entire sequence above, but to the left. Again, when breathing out, you may be able to extend the turn by a few centimetres.

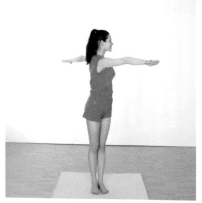

Return to the initial position.

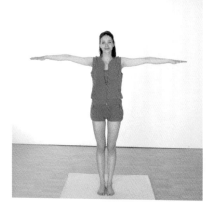

Next, lift the right arm up and bend your right arm at an angle in front of your stomach. Check that your breathing remains calm.

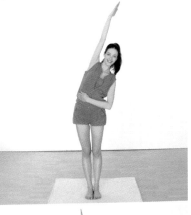

Now bend as far as you can to the left, without changing the position of your arms. Hold this posture briefly and breathe calmly in order to relax. As before, when breathing out, you may be able to extend the stretch by a few more centimetres.

Return to the initial position.

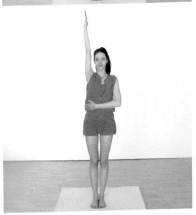

Now lift up the left arm and bend the right arm at an angle in front of the stomach. Check that you are breathing calmly.

Next, bend as far as you can to the right, without altering the position of your arms. Hold this posture briefly and breathe calmly to relax. As ever, when breathing out, you may be able to extend the stretch by a few more centimetres.

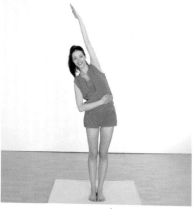

Return to the original position.

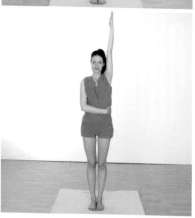

Now lift your hands and place them behind your head, folding your hands together. Again, ensure that your breathing is calm and relaxed.

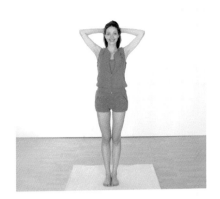

Next, bend as far as you can to the left, without altering the position of your arms. Hold this posture briefly while breathing calmly to relax. When breathing out, you may be able to extend the stretch by a few more centimetres.

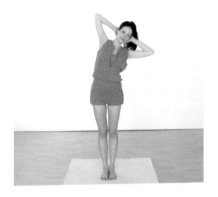

Return to the original position.

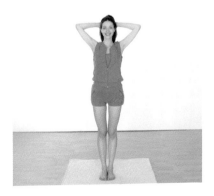

Now bend as far as you can to the right, without altering the position of your arms. Hold this posture briefly and breathe calmly to relax. As before, when breathing out, you may be able to extend the stretch by a few more centimetres.

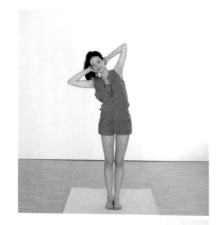

Return to the original position.

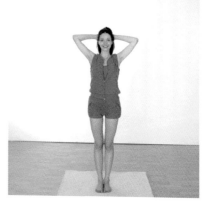

The above exercise has, purposely, been kept very short and simple. In addition, as it is carried out in a standing position, it can be done almost anywhere, whenever or wherever you are able to take a short break. Even if you only have five minutes to spare, you will soon discover just how much this exercise will relax you and refresh you simultaneously. Bodily sensations will feel better, your head will clear, and thinking will become easier.

If performed regularly, this exercise will have a relaxing effect and deepen your breathing, which will thereby improve your body's supply of oxygen. Furthermore, it will improve your flexibil-ity and improve energy flow to the merid-ians. This, in turn, will strengthen your immune system.

This exercise, borrowed from yoga, is only a very, very small part of the poten-tial offered by yoga overall. But do try it! Then, if after practising these exercises for a while, you feel like doing more, enquire about any yoga school or class in your neighbourhood.

Meditation

The word comes from the Latin *meditatio*, "to think", or "to reflect deeply". However, this does not mean just "thinking" in the usual sense of the word, i.e. when we are occupied with thinking about something. On the contrary, "meditation" actually means the complete opposite, namely being "unoccupied" with any kind of thoughts.

This is not an easy concept to grasp or to implement, especially at first. After all, we are so used to tying our concentration to our thoughts that they tend to overwhelm us as soon as we seek the inner peace of meditation. So, in order to allay this constant stream of thoughts, various techniques have to be employed:

Using a mantra – the constant repetition of a word, from the original Sanskrit *mantra*, "formula" or "saying" – is one example of a technique that is often used in order to separate one's concentration from the all-pervading stream of thoughts and divert or replace these with just the word. Depending upon the meditation tradition that is being practised, one may use as a mantra the names of gods (Hindu and Islamic traditions), famous sayings or prayer lines (Buddhist tradition), or even mere sounds or syllables that purposely have no meaning as such (from Zen Buddhism).

Nowadays, in Europe, North America, etc., affirmations or similar positive statements and expressions (such as "love", "blessings" or similar) are used as mantras. In the final analysis, counting through the Christian rosary (saying a prayer with rosary beads) is another form of a mantra meditation.

Guiding one's consciousness is another method for attaining inner calm through meditation. This method is refined particularly in the Vipassana form of meditation. By directing one's consciousness to a single process – for example, the sensation of one's breath at the tip of one's nose when breathing in and out – consciousness is withdrawn gradually, away from everything else, even stray thoughts, until inner calm is attained. Here too, there are many variations of attaining such self-observation, e.g. meditating while facing a blank white wall.

Visualisation is the third possible way of passing into a meditative state. Nearly all cultures have some form of meditation on light itself, along with spiritual images that can be conjured up. It is a process which makes it easier to separate oneself from everyday consciousness. Even such modern techniques as autogenic training can be regarded as being a form of visualisation meditation.

Rhythmic techniques include activities such as drumming and dancing and can also lead to inner calm. They form a part of most of the world's shamanisistic traditions and ceremonies and are extremely effective, leading one on a purposeful "alternative route" and removing all tensions and blockages through intense physical movement and cleansing rituals. After an initial increase in tension, there comes a sudden relaxation, which causes inner calm to be attained very rapidly. The Indian guru Osho (formerly Bhagwan Shree Rajneesh) employed similar methods especially for people with Western backgrounds and who were still unfamiliar with meditation. He found that the path through tension and relaxation gave access to meditation more quickly for such students and followers. Osho also spoke of cathartic meditations (Greek *katharsis*, "cleansing" or "purification").

Clearly, these brief descriptions do not and cannot cover the entire repertoire of meditation techniques; but that is not the subject of this book. However, the reason why meditation has a firm and valuable place in Aurum Manus® therapy is because all meditations have in common the search for that same state of "inner calm".

Inner calm

Lama Ole Nydahl, a Dane, who was trained in the tradition of Tibetan Buddhism, aptly expressed this in stating: "We are so used to occupying ourselves with the things that fill our consciousness, instead of consciousness itself."

This means that we use our everyday consciousness to observe and study everything – except ourselves. We "are" consciousness, we are "the one who is looking out through our eyes and hearing with our ears" (Ole Nydahl). But who is this really? Who are we?

This is something that nearly everyone can experience in meditation. Once we have separated our consciousness from the everyday minutiae of life and even from our own inner thoughts, nothing else remains other than "self". This may sound rather trite to those unfamiliar with meditation, but the experience of "I am who I am", which is attainable meditation, cannot be expressed adequately in words alone. It is not knowledge, but certainty. In meditation, one receives no message in the form of words. After all, that would be "thoughts" again. Instead, there emerges the certainty that one exists.

This is probably at this point that you are likely to comment, "Well, okay, but we know that anyway!" But are you certain? Can you be quite certain that "you" as such, really exist?

Modern biological science now considers that consciousness is nothing more than electrons flickering about in your brain, neurons connecting across the synapses, which cease when you die. Is there still an existence afterwards? If that is true, then where are "you" afterwards? Can you say with certainty that the scientific explanation is *not* correct? If it is right, then "you" do not exist, and you would only believe that you exist between your birth and your death – as a beautiful dream, perhaps?

From this uncertainty about our existence – the uncertainty about whether or not we are eternal beings – comes the fear of death. Surely the fear of death is, in the last instance, the mother of all fears? Yet, if you are not afraid of death – out of the certainty that you will survive anyway – what is there to be afraid of?

Maybe it helps to phrase the conviction supplied by meditation in this way: meditation supplies the certainty that "I am", the certainty that "I exist". This comes about not through a special insight, message or even a vision (among others), but simply through the repeated experience of meditation. That is the experience that we are "still here", even if there is nothing else. Even in total inner peace and calm, when consciousness is freed from all contents, we "are" – still. So we are not those mere concepts that fill our consciousness, but we are consciousness itself, we are "spirit". At this point we realise that all "things" are transitory, but consciousness is not; nor is the spirit and nor are "we". This is the "certainty of existence", which meditation bestows upon us.

In all likelihood, this does not happen in the very first meditation session. However, it does emerge certainly, gradually, with time. The gradual understanding of this certainty is the norm, and the famous and sudden experience of being "blinded by the light" is usually the exception. Even the Buddha meditated for many years, before he considered the process as being completed. The general, beneficial effects of meditation on one's life, however, will be experienced very quickly.

Benefits of meditation
The effects of meditation are those of having more inner peace in everyday life, more thoughtful actions, greater care in what we do, improved perception, diminishing fears and the disappearance of stress and tension. However, this does not mean that our ability to achieve is lessened in any way. Quite the contrary, in fact. In a calm and relaxed state, we can be much more successful in what we do; we become more efficient and things just seem to go a lot more easily.

The idea that success is only possible through effort and exertion is the idea of "doing" as contained within ancient Chinese philosophy. The concept can also be expressed as "allowing to happen", rather than "doing" or " making". In his *Tao Te*

King, the philosopher Lao Tse wrote: "The *tao* [path] remains in Not-Doing, but nothing is left undone". In essence, this is also an apt description for the "lived" meditation that can be practised in everyday life.

Meditation is one of the most important elements of Aurum Manus® therapy, as it goes to the root of all problems which lead to complaints and perceived states of all kinds. In overcoming that ancient, original fear – the fear of death or "the fear of non-existence" – many everyday fears can disappear. Along with them goes the inner sense of feeling stressed (even if one's life still includes many ostensible reasons for being stressed). As such tensions and obstructions disappear, meditation leads to holistic health of the body, soul and spirit.

Let us pause here so as to dispel any illusions. All of the above does not mean that through meditation we will no longer experience sorrow and difficulties and will henceforth float about on a cloud of bliss. Life offers us many challenges and there may be many a situation that will bring us to our knees. Loss, grief and pain are bound to remain and emotional burdens, pressing responsibilities and heavy duties will still arise.

Nevertheless, what can be changed through meditation is how we deal with all these situations. It can enhance the strength and will to master difficult and unpleasant things, and an ability to experience happiness and joy, in spite of everything. A good example of this is in the person of the Dalai Lama. Responsible for the much-oppressed people of Tibet, he certainly has more to suffer than many of us. Yet he has remained a compassionate, warm-hearted person, centred in peace and a role model for many around the world. He still derives the strength for this from meditation.

We at Aurum Manus® venture to suggest that the almost total lack of meditation in Western culture is what makes us so susceptible to all that we can best identify as the "diseases of civilisation". However "civilisation" itself is not really the problem. After all, despite the unpleasantness of these ailments and complaints, they appear to affect the Japanese far less than the West, even though they have been "civilised" for far longer. These problems are related far more to consciousness and born out of an adherence to the transitory and uncertainty about a spiritual existence. This is why Indian wise men have said that it is "ignorance which is the root evil of the world".

We hope it has become clear to our readers that meditation is one of the important possibilities whereby we can dissipate this evil.

Even in our modern and non-spiritual (for the most part) society, science has had to concede that there are some astonishing phenomena associated with meditation. Specifically, scientific research conducted with meditating people has revealed the following:

◎ Recorded brain wave patterns during meditation have shown that, in a meditative state, the brain first displays alpha rhythms and - later - theta rhythms. These correspond with the state of sleep (alpha rhythms) and the state of deep sleep (theta rhythms with a frequency of 4–7 Hz), even though the meditator is wide-awake. So maybe it is no wonder, then, that during meditation deep relaxation and regeneration are both possible in a waking state.

◎ During meditation, the absorption of oxygen in the body and the metabolism are both reduced to about 20% of their normal levels - indicating that the body's reserves are conserved.

◎ Electrical resistance increases by some 500%, which means the meditator is in a state of complete lack of fear or stress.

◎ The heart rate drops, on average by 5 beats per minute; this is also a sign of relaxation.

◎ A lower level of adrenalin is found in the blood, which also enhances a sense of calmness and relaxation.

◎ The five senses (hearing, seeing, smelling, touching and tasting) withdraw, so that there is also a reduction in the stimulation of the senses on our consciousness.

◎ Symptoms, such as tensions, lethargy, nervousness and unrest disappear.

◎ The body rids itself of toxic deposits, and the immune system is strengthened.

◎ Negative thoughts can be eliminated, and the body, spirit and soul can become healthy and whole.

A lack of agreement about the positive effects of meditation against a multitude of stress-related symptoms of complaints, such as headaches, noises in the ears, heart conditions and depression, exist even in traditional (Western) medicine. Thus even physicians and alternative practitioners recommend meditation as a self-help method.

It is said that one hour of meditation corresponds to about four hours of sleep. If we took time, in our hectic everyday lives, to engage in meditation, it would have a similar effect to several hours of sleep. We emerge from meditation with renewed vigour and vitality.

Meditation for all

Many people believe that meditating is difficult, but in reality it is the easiest thing in the world to do. Everyone can learn to meditate. The difficulty merely lies in the consistency and discipline of regularly practising it.

An important factor in overcoming this single difficulty is finding the right meditation for yourself. We live in unique times, in which so many different types of meditation techniques are potentially at our disposal, a situation that has never existed before. What was unavailable in the past, because of huge cultural and spatial separation, or was even purposely kept secret, is now offered to everyone in astonishing openness. There are some types of meditation, which we find very easy to adopt and may quickly become accustomed to using, while others remain alien and inaccessible to us in spite of much practice.

Aurum Manus® therapy does not recommend any one particular kind of meditation technique. As far as we are concerned, the result of the meditation is what is important, not the tradition or type of mediation culture from which it originates. The choice should remain what seems best for each individual, in keeping with whatever world view.

From our own experience at Aurum Manus®, we can only recommend definitely that you meditate regularly. In addition, if you are looking for the "right" type of meditation exercise that seems especially suitable – and with all your heart – you will definitely find it.

Meditation is never time lost. Indeed, it is quite the opposite; it is gaining time! If you have never had time to meditate until now, you must try it out. You will experience a state whereby you will suddenly feel that you have far more time than ever before.

Promise? Try it out...

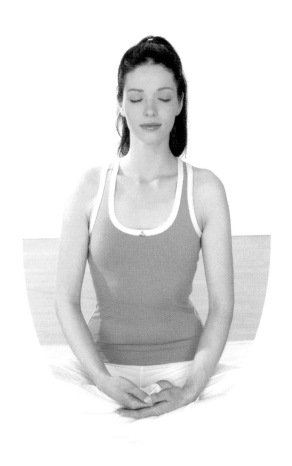

Whosever realises not-doing in doing
And doing in not-doing,
He is truly wise.

Taoist wisdom

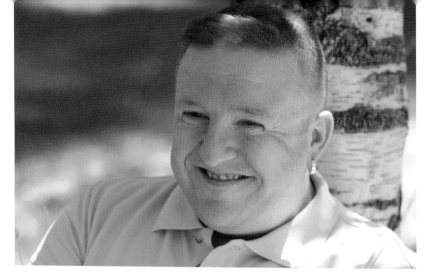

About the Author

Ricky Joe Harry Welch: born 14 September 1968, in Yakima, Washington, USA.

1988–1991: German state exams as masseur and medical pool attendant (*Bademeister*); attended the Heidelberg School of Massage, a faculty of the Heidelberg University's clinical institutes.

1988–1995: Professional attendant for various sports teams and top athletes.

1988–2005: Medical tour attendant for musicians and artistes abroad and in Germany.

1995 onwards: Freelance practitioner, presently head of the physical massage department at the US military headquarters in Heidelberg, Germany.

Special areas of activity: the development of health concepts for companies and business concerns.

◎ stress prevention
◎ post-treatment of sports injuries
◎ classic massage therapy and special massages

Since 2002, I have been giving lectures and seminars and headed training courses in Aurum Manus® therapy.

Included in my team – and among my closest colleagues – are the alternative practitioners Iris Berg from Karlsruhe-Durlach and Alfons Hubig from Heidelberg-Dossenheim.

I would like to take this opportunity to convey my heartfelt thanks to them for their co-operation and their support.

Aurum Manus®

As mentioned earlier in the book, and in some detail, prevention is absolutely indispensable and necessary for maintaining good health. However, a further reason for giving such a high priority to preventive measures is the considerable savings for those who may have private health insurance. The therapy and all the information in this book that is associated with Aurum Manus® could well reduce the risk of illness and any associated treatment costs – and this could also even include medicine/prescription costs for those in a state health system.

Aurum Manus® cures and training courses can be booked from January 2006 onward. The contact addresses of our education and therapy centres, as well as information, offers, fees and prices, and a list of licensed Aurum Manus® masseurs and masseuses may be found on our home page www.aurum-manus.de

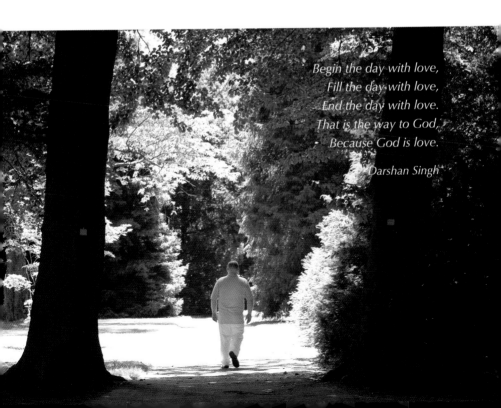

Begin the day with love,
Fill the day with love,
End the day with love.
That is the way to God,
Because God is love.

Darshan Singh

Letter from Dr. M. Lindenberger,
10.12.2000

It is estimated that there are approximately 2.7 million tinnitus sufferers among the German population, so that the annual incidence of about 340,000 new cases represents a considerable medical and environmental problem.

Hitherto, the biggest problem in both diagnosis and therapy of tinnitus has been the lack of any overall correlation or analysis of the condition that might, otherwise, form a picture of the problem. Sufferers of its acute forms can look forward to a good prognosis, provided treatment is begun early enough and is then undertaken consistently. When it comes to chronic tinnitus, however, therapeutic efforts can only really be directed at a reduction of the intensity of the symptoms and (especially) at alleviating the pressure of suffering of that patient's experience. If a return to a decent quality of life can be defined as therapeutic success, then a success rate of 80% is a reasonable calculation or estimate in such cases.

Whatever else, however, the basic and underlying principles of all tinnitus therapy have to be a low rate of complications or risk, and with a documented success rate higher than that of a mere placebo effect. Further, any decision about the actual form of a particular type of therapy for each particular patient should always take into account the specific details of date and time of the condition's onset.

In addition to therapy, tinnitus prophylaxis should be given a high priority, in order to reduce the incidence of the problem.

As a rule, the standard medical treatments, are aimed either at an improvement of the rheological situation in the area of the inner ear, or at influencing signal transmission within the hearing system.

The physical method of hyperbaric oxygen therapy leads to an enrichment of dissolved oxygen in the tissues, and thus enables a restoration the damaged functions.

Another method, tinnitus retraining therapy, leads to restoring hearing function through continuous acoustic stimulation. It is a long-term treatment but one that can sometimes, eventually, lead to a total alleviation of tinnitus.

The Aurum Manus® massage can be considered as an excellent complementary form of therapy, i.e. in addition and supplementary to the standard medical treatment of tinnitus as a therapy, Aurum Manus® incorporates aspects of massage, acupressure and relaxation therapy.

So far, experience with this therapy for tinnitus patients provides an optimistic outlook. In addition, patients who had undergone it as therapy for other reasons reported a spontaneous improvement, or even temporary (and sometimes) permanent relief from tinnitus.

Whatever the varying levels of success, some form of short- or middle-term improvement of the symptoms has been achieved by Aurum Manus® in a very considerable proportion of the tinnitus patients. In addition, the lack of side effects recommends this form of massage therapy and indicates strongly that it differs in a positive way from other medically-based treatments, such as lidocaine therapy with ECG monitoring. I would say that after a professional examination by an ear, nose and throat specialist, Aurum Manus® therapy represents a sensible addition to other procedures for a whole range of chronic tinnitus patients.

What is now needed, as a future step, is for a special patient-profile to be created from which this form of therapy can be endorsed statistically and thereby build upon its current, promising success.

Tinnitus is a problem that involves the sufferer experiencing an acoustic sensation - in effect "noise in the ear" - that occurs without there being any external source or cause of such noises being present.

In fact it is very common, being one of the most frequent of all aetiological symptoms, so that the prevalence of tinnitus as a clearly identified and specific condition involves around 0.5% of the adult population of modern industrial societies. Yet, its precise causes are still a challenge to medical science. Indeed, one often has to rely upon hypotheses to explain the aetiological problem, as a purely subjective perception of tinnitus is not easy to access through scientific and medical investigation. In turn, this also makes it difficult to assess the success rates of different forms of therapy.

Of course, it is easy enough to say that noises in the ears are symptoms of a functional disturbance within the hearing system (or in some other part of the human body). However, a detailed diagnosis by a specialist in the field of throat, nose and ear medicine is a prerequisite in order to identify the causes or influential factors of tinnitus. Only then can any treatment

be undertaken.

The period of time that has elapsed since symptoms were first experienced is also a decisive factor in the choice of therapy. Acute forms of tinnitus, which are often accompanied by loss of hearing quality, usually enjoy a good prognosis, and can even be further improved with the use of rheological, corticoid or by Hyperbaric Oxygen therapy.

The goal with any patients suffering with chronic tinnitus is a recovery of their quality of life. This explains the multitude of therapies on offer, which have some very different starting points.

The basis for a long-term, adequate treatment of a tinnitus patient is a complete diagnosis, and full explanations, which help the patient understand the possible causes and accompanying factors of his or her symptoms. Even this basic practice can, in itself, often provide a certain measure of relief for the patient. In evaluating the various types of therapy to use, the basic principle must be also be a weighing-up of the likely benefits for the patient, as well as the possible risks.

Today's standard medical treatment for most forms of chronic tinnitus include, among others, the application of

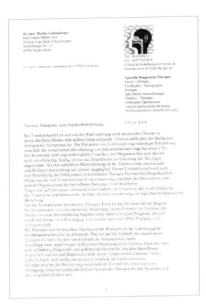

calcium antagonists, anti-arrhythmic and anti-convulsive therapy, and the use of transmitter-substances, spasmolytics and psychotropics. Tinnitus-retraining therapy (TRT) is based upon recovering use of what has become the disturbed filtering function of the hearing system. The employment of this therapy includes an accompanying verbal discussion and explanations. This is a longer-term treatment but it offers the advantage of freedom from possible side-effects of therapy relying purely upon medication.

An extension of these traditional medical therapies is the use of physical relaxation techniques. Whilst many such techniques exist, they do have in common an attempt to bring about relaxation and,

therewith, an improvement in the patient's quality of life.

The Aurum Manus® therapy incorporates relaxation by virtue of its localised application of pressure and warmth through jade crystals, reflexology foot massage, lymph drainage, and electro-acupuncture.

The experiences recorded to date on a group of more than 130 patients – all of whom had been examined previously by an ear, nose and throat specialist – indicate this form of therapy to be beneficial in alleviating chronic cases of tinnitus. It is something that promises even greater success in the future, and with the added benefit of seeming entirely free of any negative side-effects.

The Aurum Manus® Study

Aurum Manus® therapy was conducted on a group of 133 patients aged 20–75 years. All were pre-examined by an ear, nose and throat specialist.

The following post-therapy results were recorded for diagnosed tinnitus sufferers after further medical examination:

Persons treated from October 2000 to August 2001:
Total: 133 patients
Men: 82
Women: 51

problem eliminated
Improved
No change

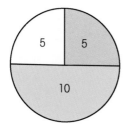

Men aged 20–40 years
20 patients
Problem eliminated: 5 persons
Improvement: 10 persons
No change: 5 persons

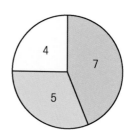

Women aged 20–40 years
16 patients
Problem eliminated: 7 persons
Improvement: 5 persons
No change: 4 persons

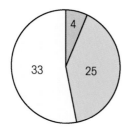

Men aged 40–75 years
62 patients
Problem eliminated: 4 persons
Improvement: 25 persons
No change: 33 persons

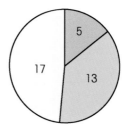

Women aged 40–75
35 patients
Problem eliminated: 5 persons
Improvement: 13 persons
No change: 17 persons

Bibliography

Ursula Dombrowsky, *Wenn Steine erzählen*, Neue Erde, Saarbrücken 2003

Michael Gienger, *Die Heilsteine der Hildegard von Bingen*, Neue Erde, Saarbrücken 2004

Michael Gienger, *The Healing Crystal First Aid Manual*, Earthdancer@Findhorn Press, 2006

Michael Gienger, *Crystal Power, Crystal Healing*, Cassell/Octopus 1998

Michael Gienger, *Die wichtigsten Heilsteine auf einen Blick* (Poster), Neue Erde, Saarbrücken 2004

Michael Gienger, *Crystal Massage for Health and Healing*, Earthdancer@Findhorn Press, 2006

Michael Gienger, *Healing Crystals, A-Z to 430 gemstones*, Earthdancer@Findhorn Press, 2005

Michael Gienger, *Heilsteine und Lebensrhythmen*, Neue Erde, Saarbrücken 2005

Michael Gienger, *Lexikon der Heilsteine*, Neue Erde, Saarbrücken 2000

Michael Gienger/Ursula Dombrowsky, *Steinheilkunde-Karten*, Neue Erde, Saarbrücken 2005

Michael Gienger/Gisela Glaser, *Salz*, Neue Erde, Saarbrücken 2003

Michael Gienger/Luna Miesala-Sellin, *Stein und Blüte*, Neue Erde, Saarbrücken 2000

Rolphe A. Grimaître, *Edelstein-Elixiere*, Neue Erde, Saarbrücken 2006

Hans Ulrich Grimm, *Die Suppe lügt*, Klett Cotta Verlag, Stuttgart 2005

Monika Grundmann, *Schönheit durch Berühren*, Neue Erde, Saarbrücken 2006

Wolfgang Maier, *Der Mondschild*, Neue Erde, Saarbrücken 2001

Barbara Newerla, *Sterne und Steine*, Neue Erde, Saarbrücken 2000

Gabriele Simon, *Erlebnismassagen für Kinder*, Neue Erde, Saarbrücken 2005

Rainer Strebel/Michael Gienger, *Die Individuelle Therapie*, AT Verlag, Baden (CH) 2005

Josef Zerluth/Michael Gienger, *Gutes Wasser*, Neue Erde, Saarbrücken 2004

Addresses and Further Information

Addresses for Aurum Manus® therapists, as well as for seminars and training, may be found on the Aurum Manus® website home page, as well as retail sources for Aurum Manus® oil cups, massage oils, etc.

Crystals are available in a wide range of dedicated retail outlets.

For further information please visit our website: www.aurum-manus.de

Ediɔion Cairn Elen

"After Elen had accomplished her wandering through the world, she placed a Cairn at the end of the Sarn Elen. Her path then led her back to the land between evening and morning. From this Cairn originated all stones that direct the way at crossroads up until today."*

(From a Celtic myth)

'Cairn Elen'* is the term used in Gaelic-speaking areas to refer to the ancient slab stones on track ways. They mark the spiritual paths, both the paths of the earth and that of knowledge.

These paths are increasingly falling into oblivion. Just as the old paths of the earth disappear under the modern asphalt streets, so also does certain ancient wisdom disappear under the data flood of modern information. For this reason, the desire and aim of the Edition Cairn Elen is to preserve ancient wisdom and link it with modern knowledge – for a flourishing future!

The Edition Cairn Elen in Neue Erde Verlag is published by Michael Gienger. The objective of the Edition is to present knowledge from research and tradition that has remained unpublished up until now. Areas of focus are nature, naturopathy and health, as well as consciousness and spiritual freedom.

Apart from current specialised literature, stories, fairytales, novels, lyric and artistic publications will also be published within the scope of Edition Cairn Elen. The knowledge thus transmitted reaches out not only to the intellect but also to the heart.

Contact
Edition Cairn Elen, Anja & Michael Gienger, Stäudach 58/1, D-72074 Tübingen,
Tel./Fax: 070 71 - 364 720, buecher@michael-gienger.de,
www.michael-gienger.de, www.steinheilkunde.de

---

[1] Celtic 'cairn' [pronounced: carn] = 'Stone' (usually placed as an intentional shaped heap of stones), 'sarn' = 'Path', 'Elen, Helen' = 'Goddess of the Roads'

* Cairn Elen: in British ancient and contemporary Celtic culture, cairns are generally intentionally heaped piles of stones, rather than an individual stone such as a boulder or standing stone.

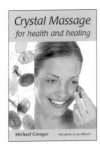

This book introduces a spectrum of massage possibilities using healing crystals. The techniques have been developed and refined by experts, and this wisdom is conveyed in simple and direct language, enhanced by photos. Any interested amateur will be amazed at the wealth of new therapeutic possibilities that open up when employing the healing power of crystals.

Michael Gienger
Crystal Massage for Health and Healing
112 Pages, full colour throughout
ISBN-13: 978-1-84409-077-8, ISBN-10: 1-84409-077-9

This is an easy-to-use A-Z guide for treating many common ailments and illnesses with the help of crystal therapy. It includes a comprehensive color appendix with photographs and short descriptions of each gemstone recommended.

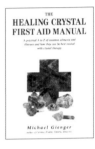

Michael Gienger
The Healing Crystals First Aid Manual
A Practical A to Z of Common Ailments and Illnesses and How They Can Be Best Treated with Crystal Therapy.
288 pages b/w + 32 color pages insert with photographs
ISBN-13: 978-1-84409-084-6, ISBN-10: 1-84409-084-1

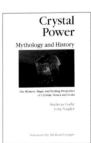

This book reveals the long- standing significance, high regard and use in therapy and healing of stones, crystals and gems – from the earliest civilizations such as Mesopotamia and Ancient Egypt, through the classical world of Greece and Rome and into medieval European cultures. In addition, there is a comprehensive Appendix, in which minerals and crystals are listed with their respective mineralogical, historical, astrological and healing properties.

Andreas Guhr, Jörg Nagler
Crystal Power: Mythology and History
The Mystery, Magic and Healing Properties
of Crystals, Stones and Gems
160 pages, full colour throughout
ISBN-13: 978-1-84409-085-3, ISBN-10: 1-84409-085-X

For further information and book catalogue contact:
Findhorn Press, 305a The Park, Forres IV36 3TE, Scottland.
Earthdancer Books is an Imprint of Findhorn Press.

tel +44 (0)1309-690582   fax +44 (0)1309-690036
info@findhornpress.com   www.earthdancer.co.uk   www.findhornpress.com

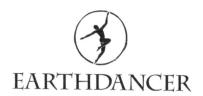

EARTHDANCER

A FINDHORN PRESS IMPRINT